# From Gene to Function: CEACAM1's Role in Maintaining Glucose Homeostasis

Jacksin

# Table of Contents

**Carcinoembryonic Antigen-Related Cell Adhesion Molecule1 (CEACAM1)**

CEACAM1 is a transmembrane glycoprotein that is expressed in a variety of cells including endothelial, immune, and epithelial cells of most tissues. Among the insulin target tissues, CEACAM1 is expressed predominantly in the liver, and to a lower extend in the adipose tissue, but it is not expressed in the skeletal muscle [1]. CEACAM1 is a member of the immunoglobulin (Ig) superfamily; and it is remarkably well conserved among the different species [2]. Various functions have been attributed to CEACAM1, including angiogenesis and vasculogenesis [3]; tumor suppression [4, 5]; cell-cell interaction [4]; and anti-inflammation in activated immune cells [6]. CEACAM1 also plays an important role in promoting insulin function by sustaining hepatic insulin clearance to prevent hyperinsulinemia and hepatic lipogenesis [2, 7].

Ceacam1 gene is alternatively spliced into 2 isoforms. The cytoplasmic domain of its long isoform has two Immunoreceptor Tyrosine-based Inhibitory Motifs (ITIMs) (SHP-1, and SHP-2) [8]. When CEACAM1 is phosphorylated by the insulin receptor tyrosine kinase in response to insulin, it binds to SHP-2 to sequester it away from binding IRS-1 [9]. This causes an increase in IRS-1 phosphorylation and activation of its downstream targets such as elements in the PI3K/Akt/eNOS pathway [9]. This suggests that in endothelial cells, CEACAM1 plays an important role in maintaining endothelial cell autonomous effects by promoting nitric oxide bioavailability.

Moreover, upon its phosphorylation by vascular endothelial growth factor receptor (VEGFR), CEACAM1binds to SHP-2 to cause phosphorylation of downstream

Src kinase which results in Src kinase inactivation [3]. Usually, activated Src kinase phosphorylates intercellular adhesion molecule 1 (ICAM1) and increases leukocyte-endothelial interaction worsening the vascular morphology [3]. Therefore, binding of SHP-2 to phosphorylated CEACAM1 decreases endothelial adhesion to leukocytes [3]. Additionally, binding of phosphorylated CEACAM1 to SHP-2 conveys inhibitory signals to the T-cell receptor, B-cell receptor, and epithelial growth factor [8]. This demonstrates anti-inflammatory properties of the long isoform of CEACAM1 [8].

**Insulin**

The discovery of insulin goes back to 1921 [10]. Insulin is synthesized as pre-proinsulin then processed to proinsulin which is converted to insulin and C-peptide [11]. When pancreatic beta-cells are stimulated, insulin is secreted by exocytosis in a pulsatile manner [12]. In order to maintain physiologic insulin levels, a balance between insulin secretion and insulin clearance needs to be achieved. Insulin is transported rapidly to the liver via the portal vein where its half-life is about 3-5 minutes. Under normal physiologic conditions, secreted insulin reaching the hepatocytes through fenestrae in liver capillaries undergoes clearance (by ~ 80%) during its first pass. Unprocessed insulin is delivered to the systemic circulation to exert its action in insulin targeted tissues. Unlike the liver's capillaries, capillaries of extra-hepatic insulin target tissues lack fenestration and the passage of insulin is tightly controlled by endothelial cells lining their vasculature [12].

Insulin exerts its action by binding to cell surface receptor [13]. The insulin receptor has two subunits, an extracellular alpha subunit which binds to the hormone, and a beta subunit which bears a tyrosine-specific protein kinase in its cytoplasmic tail [13].

Activation of this tyrosine kinase by insulin binding initiates insulin's action on glucose,

lipid, and protein metabolism [13]. At the cellular level, insulin action is modulated by

altered binding to and activation of this tyrosine kinase, or by changes in the number of

insulin receptors. At the whole organism level, insulin sensitivity is affected by a

multitude of factors ranging from genetic variants of the structure and function of insulin

receptor, to sedentary lifestyle and unhealthy eating habits [7].

Insulin plays a critical role in vascular homeostasis and understanding the actions

of insulin on the vasculature is of high importance [14]. Studies on endothelial insulin

receptor and apolipoprotein E knockout (EIRAKO) mice provided evidence that loss of

insulin signaling in the endothelium accelerates atherosclerosis in the EIRAKO mice

compared with their littermate apolipoprotein E knockout mice control, in spite of

differences in whole-body insulin sensitivity, plasma lipids, or glucose tolerance between

the two groups [15]. This suggests that atherosclerosis can be the result of the loss of

insulin action in vascular endothelial cells [15]. Several reports have established the

pleiotropic actions of insulin in vascular endothelium such as generating nitric oxide,

preventing inflammation, and decreasing monocyte recruitment [16]. This is regulated, at

least in part, by the forkhead protein FOXO1, a transcription factor that undergoes

inactivation and nuclear exclusion upon its phosphorylation by AKT [16]. Oxidative

stress in endothelial cells is one factor that activates FOXO1 resulting in up-regulation of

inducible nitric oxide synthase (iNOS) that leads to oxidative modifications of LDL and endothelial nitric oxide synthase dysfunction [17]. This indicates that FOXO1 activation promotes generation of peroxynitrite and suppresses vascular homeostasis [17].

CEACAM1 is a shared substrate of insulin and VEGF receptors. Thus, studying VEGF signaling in relation to CEACAM1 is expected to advance our understanding of the molecular transduction pathways leading to chronic diseases such as atherosclerosis. Moreover, given that atherosclerosis is well associated with endothelium injury, it is reasonable to link it to endothelial-cell insulin resistance and defective VEGF signaling.

**Vascular Endothelial Growth Factor (VEGF)**

The angiogenic cytokine, VEGF is predominantly expressed in endothelial cells, and is produced by other cells such as fibroblasts, neutrophils, and macrophages to a lower extent [18]. While many factors have been reported to induce VEGF production such as cytokines, nitric oxide, and oncogenes [18], hypoxia is the most potent stimulus for VEGF expression. The downstream signaling cascades of VEGF receptor (VEGFR) activation have been delineated, while the mechanisms involved in the production of VEGF are still elusive.

It has been established that CEACAM1 is an effector of VEGF [19]. VEGF-A is one of the most important factors mediating angiogenesis; VEGF-A binds to and activates both VEGF-R1 and VEGF-R2 [20]. However, VEGF-A is complexed with VEGF-R2 to maintain its expression and downstream signal transduction events [20]. VEGF receptors work via both AKT and nuclear factor-κB (NF-κB) pathways to promote angiogenesis. Additionally, there is evidence that VEGF is regulated by NF-κB [18] and recent studies reported that angiogenesis inhibition is associated to NF-κB activation

[21]. Pro-inflammatory cytokines such as TNFα and IL-6 can activate NF-κB. These stimuli elevate IκB kinases which phosphorylate the main inhibitor, IκBα. This phosphorylation results in degradation of IκBα and leads to the translocation of the NF-κB complex to the nucleus where it binds to κB enhancers to activate transcription [21]. Altered signaling of CEACAM1-dependent pathways disrupts the endothelial cell response to insulin and VEGF and contributes to atherosclerosis predisposition partly through activation of NF-κB.

**Compromised Vasodilation**

Endothelial cells produce nitric oxide (NO) by metabolizing L-arginine via the endothelial nitric oxide synthase (eNOS) [22]. Basally, NO is a potent vasodilator and has anti-atherogenic effects [23]; as well as it regulates vasomotor tone and maintains vascular lining [24]. Alternations to eNOS activity and NO bioavailability result in compromised vasodilation which can be an independent predictor of atherosclerosis [25]. Moreover, compromised vasoconstriction is characterized by an increased endothelin-1 (ET-1) production. Endothelin-1 works through its receptors, EtR-A and EtR-B. EtR-A signals vasoconstriction while EtR-B elicits vasodilation through the release of NO. Therefore, increased production of ET-1 and expression of the ratio of EtR-A/EtR-B indicates increased vasoconstriction and fibrogenesis [26].

Consistent with CEACAM1 being a substrate of both insulin and VEGF receptors, mice with global deletion of *Ceacam1* gene (*Cc1*$^{-/-}$) exhibited reduced endothelial cell response to VEGF and increased basal endothelial permeability [9]. In order to maintain normal eNOS activity and NO production, insulin and VEGF activation of AKT are required. CEACAM1 plays an important role in AKT/eNOS activation in response to insulin in endothelial cells. This was demonstrated in cultured bovine aortic endothelial cells with siRNA-mediated downregulation of bovine CEACAM1 [9]. Western analysis showed higher expression of VCAM-1 and pIκb-α levels and lower AKT/eNOS activation [9]. This positions CEACAM1 as a regulator of AKT1 activation of eNOS that is a vital step in mediating endothelial homeostasis. This also demonstrates that CEACAM1 maintains endothelial cell autonomous mechanisms involved in vascular morphology and NO production in aortae [9].

**Inflammation and Fibrosis**

Acute inflammation starts as a healthy response to repair a site of injury. This response is presented as redness or swelling and is termed acute phase response [27]. Inflamed sites attract leukocytes as a defense reaction to recruit inflammatory mediators resulting in activation of blood vessel endothelium to increase permeability of cytokines initiating tissue healing [28]. When inflammation is prolonged or repeated, it leads to altered mechanical properties of organs and ends in dysfunction; this is termed chronic inflammation. This type of inflammation is an important trigger for fibrosis development. Many of the classical proinflammatory cytokines such as IL-6, IL-1β, and TNF-α are also profibrotic [29]. Inflammation and fibrosis are the hallmarks of a wide range of diseases including atherosclerosis and nonalcoholic steatohepatitis (NASH). Importantly, chronic inflammation contributes to the emergence of pathological conditions such as obesity, diabetes, cancer [30], and age-related diseases [31].

Systemic chronic inflammation is associated with disturbance of tissue function or homeostatic imbalance. There are well established molecular and cellular mechanisms of inflammation-related diseases. Atherosclerosis-related inflammation is mediated by a number of markers including C - reactive protein, IL-6, adhesion molecules, and matrix metalloproteinase [32, 33]. Many reports have demonstrated that these markers could be used to detect the vulnerability of atherosclerotic plaques [34-36]. Moreover, major inflammatory signaling pathways involved in atherosclerosis development have been well investigated and provided better understanding of the pathogenesis of this disease. These signaling pathways are toll-like receptor 4 (TLR4) signaling, NF-κB signaling, and the Janus kinase (JAK) - signal transducer and activator of transcription (STAT) signaling. Interestingly, NASH and atherosclerosis could share a common etiology and hence a shared inflammatory signaling pathway [37, 38]. In fact, many reports showed that cytokines such as IL-6 and TNF-α contribute to hepatic insulin resistance and could activate JAK-STAT3 and NF-κB signaling pathways to cause pro-inflammation and pro-fibrogenesis in NASH [39].

Immunological regulation and anti-inflammatory therapies could prevent the occurrence of atherosclerosis and NASH by preventing chronic organ failure and fibrosis. Proven clinical measures that aim at suppressing inflammation could be a novel breakthrough to treat fibro-inflammatory diseases. However, a high degree of redundancy is present in factors inducing fibrosis. Hindering a group of profibrotic cytokines may lead to a reciprocal upregulation of another group of profibrotic factors. In fact, some profibrotic cytokines have important anti-inflammatory properties such as IL-4 and IL-13 [40]. Hence, targeting the right combination of factors for prevention of fibro-inflammatory diseases would depend on the stage of the disease and the inflammatory milieu present in the tissue.

**Atherosclerosis**

Atherosclerosis remains a leading cause of death in the United States and worldwide [41]. Individuals with metabolic syndrome are more susceptible to developing atherosclerosis [41]. Atherosclerosis is a progressive inflammatory disease that involves the loss of vascular homeostasis [42]. This disease is characterized by accumulation of fat in aortic wall and subsequent complex inflammatory and fibro-proliferative response to endothelium damage [42]. The endothelium is responsible for regulating vascular permeability. Injury to the vascular endothelium causes the release of cell surface adhesion molecules which results in changes to the endothelial cell morphology and the subsequent increase in permeability of lipids and fluids to the intimal endothelium [43]. Several reports have demonstrated the role of altered vascular permeability in aggravating a number of diseases including atherosclerosis [44, 45]. Endothelial dysfunction has been shown to be one of the important pathological events that cause atherosclerosis by a combination of metabolic and inflammatory derangements [46]. Endothelial cell injury allows more inflammatory molecules into the vessel wall. There is increasing evidence for altered expression of endothelial cell adhesion molecules in inflammation [47].

During hypoxia and atherosclerosis, CEACAM1 is upregulated to mediate the remodeling of the endothelial barrier function. This suggests a role for CEACAM1 in vascular homeostasis [48]. Moreover, CEACAM1 expression is increased in activated endothelium of atherosclerotic plaques in *ApoE*$^{-/-}$ aortae [3]. This demonstrates that

CEACAM1 is required for endothelial cell function.  Furthermore, endothelial-cell

specific overexpression of CEACAM1 in mice improved wrapping of the endothelial

barrier by pericytes which allows endothelial cells to differentiate and form vascular

branches [49]. This also suggests that CEACAM1 facilitates heterotypic adhesion

between endothelial cells and accessory cells such as pericytes [19].

Atherosclerosis is a lipoprotein-driven disease that leads to plaque formation at

areas of increased shear stress of arterial blood vessels through intimal inflammation,

necrosis, and fibrosis [50]. Being an essential component of the cell membrane,

cholesterol is required by all mammalian cells [51]. Moreover, cholesterol is a key

component of arterial plaques; in fact, elevated levels of low density lipoprotein (LDL)

cholesterol and Apolipoprotein B100 (ApoB100) are associated with a higher risk for

atherosclerotic cardiovascular conditions [52].  Concerning the size of LDL contributing

to the development of atherosclerosis, small dense LDL particles and oxidized LDL are

highly associated with atherosclerosis [53]. In fact, circulating oxidized LDL is an

identifying marker for patients with coronary artery disease [54]. Thus far, LDL lowering

drugs and insulin sensitizers are the most effective therapies against atherosclerotic

cardiovascular disease [55]. However, there remains some genetic variability among

patients which is due to the heterogeneity of metabolic diseases [56]. Therefore, targeting

other aspects of the disease such as the inflammatory and fibrotic processes could present

a novel therapeutic modality. In fact, our studies will argue that inducing CEACAM1

expression could potentially be an effective therapeutic alternative.

**Lipids**

Obesity, particularly excess visceral fat accumulation, is the major factor driving

the epidemic of type 2 diabetes and cardiovascular diseases [23]. It is widely accepted

among the scientific and medical scholars that accumulation of fat in tissues such as liver,

muscle, heart, and aorta is associated with insulin resistance [57]. The development of

insulin resistance is related to the deleterious effects of excess tissue and plasma fatty

acids accumulation, which occurs from de novo lipogenesis and the imbalance of energy

intake and energy consumption [23]. Fatty acids (FA) play a pivotal role in the etiology

of the metabolic syndrome by serving as cellular signaling molecules [58]. Long-chain

fatty acids are crucial constituents of membrane lipids and a major source of energy [58].

Oxidation of long chain fatty acids such as palmitate requires the transport of FA-CoA

into the mitochondria by carnitine palmitoyltransferase (CPT-1). Mitochondrial fatty acid

oxidation is also regulated by malonyl-CoA, which inhibits the function of CPT-1 [51,

59]. Malonyl-CoA inhibition of CPT-1 provides an important mechanism of two

divergent pathways: fatty acid synthesis and fatty acid oxidation [58].

CEACAM1 has been shown to regulate fatty acid $\beta$-oxidation in the liver during

the fasting-refeeding transition [60, 61]. At fasting, metabolism shifts from glycolysis to

lipolysis and the white adipose tissue starts releasing free fatty acids (FFA) into the liver

to undergo beta-oxidation. This mechanism is mediated by activation of peroxisome

proliferator-activated receptor $\alpha$ (PPAR$\alpha$), a transcription factor that induces the

expression of genes involved in $\beta$-oxidation [62]. In the first few hours of refeeding (~ 8

hours), hepatic $\beta$-oxidation gradually stops with the stepwise recovery of malonyl-CoA that inhibits CPT-1 (the enzyme responsible for fatty acids translocation to the mitochondria to be oxidized). This on-and-off break on β-oxidation is mediated by the coordinated activation of PPARα with the pulsatile release of insulin during the early hours of refeeding. Whereas PPARα suppresses CEACAM1 expression when insulin is low, pulsatile insulin elevates CEACAM1 expression and its phosphorylation to increase its binding to and downregulation of the activity of fatty acid synthase (FASN), a lipogenic enzyme that catalyzes the conversion of malonyl-CoA to palmitic acid [2, 63]. This demonstrates the crucial role of CEACAM1 in regulating both insulin and fatty acid homeostasis [64, 65].

**Hyperinsulinemia and Insulin Resistance**

Insulin mediates a cascade of events during the glucose-lipid crosstalk. In response to high levels of blood glucose, insulin promotes glucose storage as glycogen in the liver, and glucose uptake in muscle and adipose tissue [66]. In adipocytes, insulin also promotes triglyceride uptake and storage, and inhibits lipolysis. Lipid buildup (referred to as lipotoxicity) in muscle and liver alters insulin action to contribute to insulin resistance and hyperglycemia [67]. Redistribution of free fatty acids to adipose tissue through activation of peroxisome proliferator-activated receptor γ (PPARγ) by agonists [68] has been the major intervention for the treatment of type 2 diabetes mellitus and in part nonalcoholic fatty liver disease (NAFLD).

Insulin action is regulated by the concentration of circulating insulin, which is a balance between insulin secretion from pancreatic β-cells and hepatic insulin clearance [69, 70]. Work on CEACAM1 shed light on its novel role in maintaining insulin sensitivity by promoting insulin clearance in the liver [2]. Moreover, extensive research using various CEACAM1 mouse models of both loss-of-function and gain-of-function validated the notion that impaired ability to clear insulin causes chronic hyperinsulinemia, which results in peripheral insulin resistance [71, 72]. However, clinical studies have challenged the cause-effect relationship between impaired insulin clearance and insulin resistance and whether insulin resistance precedes or follows hyperinsulinemia remains under investigation. Insulin also plays a critical role in lipid metabolism and vascular homeostasis.

Implications of the role of insulin resistance in the development of both atherosclerosis and NAFLD is well accepted [23, 73]. At the cellular level, it has been confirmed that loss of insulin action in vascular endothelial cells could accelerate cardiovascular complications [15]. In fact, insulin resistance is the endothelium impairs NO bioavailability and increases redox imbalance [14]. Thus, intact insulin signaling in the endothelium is essential to maintain normal cellular function. In NAFLD, insulin resistance is present at the level of the muscle, liver and adipose tissue [74]. Insulin resistance triggers ectopic fat accumulation partly due to increased transcription of lipogenic genes by the master regulator of lipogenesis, sterol regulatory element-binding protein 1c (SREBP-1c). This leads to lipotoxicity that induced a pro-inflammatory state along with increased production of fibrogenic mediators causing hepatic fibrosis.

**Nonalcoholic Fatty Liver Disease/NAFLD and Nonalcoholic Steatohepatitis/NASH**

Metabolic syndrome is a cluster of metabolic abnormalities including visceral obesity, dyslipidemia, and hypertension [75]. Importantly, metabolic syndrome is a leading cause of mortality and morbidity in developed countries [76]. Mounting

epidemiological evidence supports the notion that metabolic syndrome is linked with

NAFLD and its progressive form, NASH [77]. NASH is the most common chronic liver

disorder worldwide [73, 78], approximately 30% of adults in industrialized countries

have NAFLD, and 20% of these cases are classified as NASH [73, 79]. Moreover, the

prevalence of NAFLD is expected to increase by 21% in the next 15 years, with parallel

increase in NASH and liver related diseases [80].

NASH pathologies include macrosteatosis as well as lobular inflammation [81],

hepatocellular injury, apoptosis, and hepatic bridging fibrosis [82-84]. Hepatic sinusoidal

endothelial cells play a key role in the progression of liver fibrosis and cirrhosis [85].

Historically, insulin resistance has been implicated in driving NAFLD [76]. Reduction in

CEACAM1 expression causes insulin resistance [64] and liver injury [86]. Various

studies on mice with global null deletion of the *Ceacam1* gene ($Cc1^{-/-}$) [87], mice with

liver-specific inactivation of CEACAM1 [71] and mice with liver-specific deletion of the

*Ceacam1* gene [72] exhibited impairment of insulin clearance, followed by

hyperinsulinemia and insulin resistance. Additionally, *Ceacam1* mutant mice showed

features of benign NAFLD with first stages of fibrosis when fed a regular diet, and

progressive NASH with more robust fibrosis upon high fat feeding [88, 89]. These

studies demonstrated that reduced hepatic CEACAM1 provides a molecular mechanism

for NASH. Together, altered CEACAM1-signaling pathways disrupt insulin action and

contribute to the development of NASH.

**References**

1.      Heinrich, G., et al., *Loss of Hepatic CEACAM1: A Unifying Mechanism Linking Insulin Resistance to Obesity and Non-Alcoholic Fatty Liver Disease.* Front Endocrinol (Lausanne), 2017. 8: p. 8.

2.      Najjar, S.M., *Regulation of insulin action by CEACAM1.* Trends Endocrinol Metab, 2002. 13(6): p. 240-5.

3.      Ghavampour, S., et al., *Endothelial barrier function is differentially regulated by CEACAM1-mediated signaling.* FASEB J, 2018. 32(10): p. 5612-5625.

4.      Obrink, B., *CEA adhesion molecules: multifunctional proteins with signal-regulatory properties.* Curr Opin Cell Biol, 1997. 9(5): p. 616-26.

5.      Liu, J., et al., *Loss of Ceacam1 promotes prostate cancer progression in Pten haploinsufficient male mice.* Metabolism, 2020. 107: p. 154215.

6.      Gray-Owen, S.D. and R.S. Blumberg, *CEACAM1: contact-dependent control of immunity.* Nat Rev Immunol, 2006. 6(6): p. 433-46.

7.      Bergman, R.N., et al., *Hypothesis: Role of Reduced Hepatic Insulin Clearance in the Pathogenesis of Type 2 Diabetes.* Diabetes, 2019. 68(9): p. 1709-1716.

8.      Gu, A., et al., *Generation of Human CEACAM1 Transgenic Mice and Binding of Neisseria Opa Protein to Their Neutrophils.* Plos One, 2010. 5(4).

9.      Najjar, S.M., et al., *Ceacam1 deletion causes vascular alterations in large vessels.* Am J Physiol Endocrinol Metab, 2013. 305(4): p. E519-29.

10.     Rosenfeld, L., *Insulin: Discovery and controversy.* Clinical Chemistry, 2002. 48(12): p. 2270-2288.

11.	Fu, Z., E.R. Gilbert, and D. Liu, *Regulation of insulin synthesis and secretion and pancreatic Beta-cell dysfunction in diabetes.* Curr Diabetes Rev, 2013. 9(1): p. 25-53.

12.	Najjar, S.M. and G. Perdomo, *Hepatic Insulin Clearance: Mechanism and Physiology.* Physiology, 2019. 34(3): p. 198-215.

13.	Kahn, C.R., *The Molecular Mechanism of Insulin Action.* Annual Review of Medicine, 1985. 36: p. 429-451.

14.	Rajwani, A., R.M. Cubbon, and S.B. Wheatcroft, *Cell-specific insulin resistance: implications for atherosclerosis.* Diabetes Metab Res Rev, 2012. 28(8): p. 627-34.

15.	Rask-Madsen, C., et al., *Loss of insulin signaling in vascular endothelial cells accelerates atherosclerosis in apolipoprotein E null mice.* Cell Metab, 2010. 11(5): p. 379-89.

16.	Tsuchiya, K., et al., *FoxOs integrate pleiotropic actions of insulin in vascular endothelium to protect mice from atherosclerosis.* Cell Metab, 2012. 15(3): p. 372-81.

17.	Tanaka, J., et al., *Foxo1 links hyperglycemia to LDL oxidation and endothelial nitric oxide synthase dysfunction in vascular endothelial cells.* Diabetes, 2009. 58(10): p. 2344-54.

18.	Kiriakidis, S., et al., *VEGF expression in human macrophages is NF-kappaB-dependent: studies using adenoviruses expressing the endogenous NF-kappaB inhibitor IkappaBalpha and a kinase-defective form of the IkappaB kinase 2.* J Cell Sci, 2003. 116(Pt 4): p. 665-74.

19.     Wagener, C. and S. Ergun, *Angiogenic properties of the carcinoembryonic antigen-related cell adhesion molecule 1.* Exp Cell Res, 2000. 261(1): p. 19-24.

20.     E, G., et al., *Endogenous vascular endothelial growth factor-A (VEGF-A) maintains endothelial cell homeostasis by regulating VEGF receptor-2 transcription.* J Biol Chem, 2012. 287(5): p. 3029-41.

21.     Tabruyn, S.P. and A.W. Griffioen, *NF-kappa B: a new player in angiostatic therapy.* Angiogenesis, 2008. 11(1): p. 101-6.

22.     Gimbrone, M.A., Jr. and G. Garcia-Cardena, *Endothelial Cell Dysfunction and the Pathobiology of Atherosclerosis.* Circ Res, 2016. 118(4): p. 620-36.

23.     Di Pino, A. and R.A. DeFronzo, *Insulin Resistance and Atherosclerosis: Implications for Insulin-Sensitizing Agents.* Endocr Rev, 2019. 40(6): p. 1447-1467.

24.     Tousoulis, D., et al., *The role of nitric oxide on endothelial function.* Curr Vasc Pharmacol, 2012. 10(1): p. 4-18.

25.     Davignon, J. and P. Ganz, *Role of endothelial dysfunction in atherosclerosis.* Circulation, 2004. 109(23 Suppl 1): p. III27-32.

26.     Fan, J.L., et al., *Role of endothelin-1 in atherosclerosis.* Atherosclerosis V: The Fifth Saratoga Conference, 2000. 902: p. 84-94.

27.     Benjamin, E.J., et al., *Heart Disease and Stroke Statistics-2017 Update: A Report From the American Heart Association.* Circulation, 2017. 135(10): p. e146-e603.

28.     Ross, R., *The pathogenesis of atherosclerosis: a perspective for the 1990s.* Nature, 1993. 362(6423): p. 801-9.

29.  Galkina, E. and K. Ley, *Immune and inflammatory mechanisms of atherosclerosis (*)*. Annu Rev Immunol, 2009. 27: p. 165-97.

30.  Frank, P.G. and M.P. Lisanti, *ICAM-1: role in inflammation and in the regulation of vascular permeability*. Am J Physiol Heart Circ Physiol, 2008. 295(3): p. H926-H927.

31.  Jeong, J., et al., *Soluble RAGE attenuates AngII-induced endothelial hyperpermeability by disrupting HMGB1-mediated crosstalk between AT1R and RAGE*. Exp Mol Med, 2019. 51(9): p. 113.

32.  Varghese, J.F., R. Patel, and U.C.S. Yadav, *Novel insights in the metabolic syndrome-induced oxidative stress and inflammation-mediated atherosclerosis*. Curr Cardiol Rev, 2017.

33.  Reglero-Real, N., et al., *Endothelial Cell Junctional Adhesion Molecules: Role and Regulation of Expression in Inflammation*. Arterioscler Thromb Vasc Biol, 2016. 36(10): p. 2048-2057.

34.  Rueckschloss, U., S. Kuerten, and S. Ergun, *The role of CEA-related cell adhesion molecule-1 (CEACAM1) in vascular homeostasis*. Histochem Cell Biol, 2016. 146(6): p. 657-671.

35.  Gerstel, D., et al., *CEACAM1 creates a pro-angiogenic tumor microenvironment that supports tumor vessel maturation*. Oncogene, 2011. 30(41): p. 4275-4288.

36.  Usman, A., et al., *From Lipid Retention to Immune-Mediate Inflammation and Associated Angiogenesis in the Pathogenesis of Atherosclerosis*. J Atheroscler Thromb, 2015. 22(8): p. 739-49.

37.     Schulze, P.C., K. Drosatos, and I.J. Goldberg, *Lipid Use and Misuse by the Heart.* Circulation Research, 2016. 118(11): p. 1736-1751.

38.     Linton, M.R.F., et al., *The Role of Lipids and Lipoproteins in Atherosclerosis*, in *Endotext*, K.R. Feingold, et al., Editors. 2000: South Dartmouth (MA).

39.     Sakurai, T., et al., *Measurement of lipoprotein particle sizes using dynamic light scattering.* Ann Clin Biochem, 2010. 47(Pt 5): p. 476-81.

40.     Chen, Q., et al., *Association of anti-oxidized LDL and candidate genes with severity of coronary stenosis in the Women's Ischemia Syndrome Evaluation study.* J Lipid Res, 2011. 52(4): p. 801-7.

41.     Tabas, I., K.J. Williams, and J. Boren, *Subendothelial lipoprotein retention as the initiating process in atherosclerosis - Update and therapeutic implications.* Circulation, 2007. 116(16): p. 1832-1844.

42.     Neeland, I.J., P. Poirier, and J.P. Despres, *Cardiovascular and Metabolic Heterogeneity of Obesity: Clinical Challenges and Implications for Management.* Circulation, 2018. 137(13): p. 1391-1406.

43.     Petersen, K.F. and G.I. Shulman, *Etiology of insulin resistance.* American Journal of Medicine, 2006. 119(5): p. 10s-16s.

44.     Wakil, S.J. and L.A. Abu-Elheiga, *Fatty acid metabolism: target for metabolic syndrome.* Journal of Lipid Research, 2009. 50: p. S138-S143.

45.     Leone, T.C., C.J. Weinheimer, and D.P. Kelly, *A critical role for the peroxisome proliferator-activated receptor alpha (PPARalpha) in the cellular fasting response:*

*the PPARalpha-null mouse as a model of fatty acid oxidation disorders.* Proc Natl Acad Sci U S A, 1999. 96(13): p. 7473-8.

46.     Ramakrishnan, S.K., et al., *PPARalpha (Peroxisome Proliferator-activated Receptor alpha) Activation Reduces Hepatic CEACAM1 Protein Expression to Regulate Fatty Acid Oxidation during Fasting-refeeding Transition.* J Biol Chem, 2016. 291(15): p. 8121-9.

47.     Evans, R.M., G.D. Barish, and Y.X. Wang, *PPARs and the complex journey to obesity.* Nat Med, 2004. 10(4): p. 355-61.

48.     Kersten, S., et al., *Peroxisome proliferator-activated receptor alpha mediates the adaptive response to fasting.* J Clin Invest, 1999. 103(11): p. 1489-98.

49.     Najjar, S.M., et al., *Insulin acutely decreases hepatic fatty acid synthase activity.* Cell Metab, 2005. 2(1): p. 43-53.

50.     Najjar, S.M. and G. Perdomo, *Hepatic Insulin Clearance: Mechanism and Physiology.* Physiology (Bethesda), 2019. 34(3): p. 198-215.

51.     Najjar, S.M., *The Lipogenic Effect of Insulin Revisited*, in *Hepatic De Novo Lipogenesis and Regulation of Metabolism*, J.M. Ntambi, Editor. 2016, Springer International Publishing: Cham. p. 285-295.

52.     Jia, G., V.G. DeMarco, and J.R. Sowers, *Insulin resistance and hyperinsulinaemia in diabetic cardiomyopathy.* Nat Rev Endocrinol, 2016. 12(3): p. 144-53.

53.     Chen, W., E. Balland, and M.A. Cowley, *Hypothalamic Insulin Resistance in Obesity: Effects on Glucose Homeostasis.* Neuroendocrinology, 2017. 104(4): p. 364-381.

54.     Hong, F., et al., *PPARs as Nuclear Receptors for Nutrient and Energy Metabolism.* Molecules, 2019. 24(14).

55.     Tokarz, V.L., P.E. MacDonald, and A. Klip, *The cell biology of systemic insulin function.* J Cell Biol, 2018. 217(7): p. 2273-2289.

56.     Thomas, D.D., et al., *Hyperinsulinemia: An Early Indicator of Metabolic Dysfunction.* J Endocr Soc, 2019. 3(9): p. 1727-1747.

57.     Poy, M.N., et al., *CEACAM1 regulates insulin clearance in liver.* Nat Genet, 2002. 30(3): p. 270-6.

58.     Ghadieh, H.E., et al., *Hyperinsulinemia drives hepatic insulin resistance in male mice with liver-specific Ceacam1 deletion independently of lipolysis.* Metabolism, 2019. 93: p. 33-43.

59.     Watt, M.J., et al., *The Liver as an Endocrine Organ-Linking NAFLD and Insulin Resistance.* Endocr Rev, 2019. 40(5): p. 1367-1393.

60.     Gastaldelli, A. and K. Cusi, *From NASH to diabetes and from diabetes to NASH: Mechanisms and treatment options.* JHEP Rep, 2019. 1(4): p. 312-328.

61.     Zimmet, P., et al., *Etiology of the Metabolic Syndrome: Potential role of insulin resistance, leptin resistance, and other players.* The Metabolic Syndrome X, 1999. 892: p. 25-44.

62.     Perry, R.J., et al., *The role of hepatic lipids in hepatic insulin resistance and type 2 diabetes.* Nature, 2014. 510(7503): p. 84-91.

63.    Najjar, S.M. and L. Russo, *CEACAM1 loss links inflammation to insulin resistance in obesity and non-alcoholic steatohepatitis (NASH)*. Semin Immunopathol, 2014. 36(1): p. 55-71.

64.    Jennings, J., C. Faselis, and M.D. Yao, *NAFLD-NASH: An Under-Recognized Epidemic*. Curr Vasc Pharmacol, 2018. 16(3): p. 209-213.

65.    Younossi, Z.M., et al., *Global Epidemiology of Nonalcoholic Fatty Liver Disease-Meta-Analytic Assessment of Prevalence, Incidence, and Outcomes*. Hepatology, 2016. 64(1): p. 73-84.

66.    Estes, C., et al., *Modeling the epidemic of nonalcoholic fatty liver disease demonstrates an exponential increase in burden of disease*. Hepatology, 2018. 67(1): p. 123-133.

67.    Di Conza, G. and P.C. Ho, *ER Stress Responses: An Emerging Modulator for Innate Immunity*. Cells, 2020. 9(3).

68.    Jung, K.Y., et al., *Nonalcoholic steatohepatitis associated with metabolic syndrome: relationship to insulin resistance and liver histology*. J Clin Gastroenterol, 2014. 48(10): p. 883-8.

69.    Czaja, A.J., *Hepatic inflammation and progressive liver fibrosis in chronic liver disease*. World J Gastroenterol, 2014. 20(10): p. 2515-32.

70.    Rozpedek, W., et al., *The Role of the PERK/eIF2alpha/ATF4/CHOP Signaling Pathway in Tumor Progression During Endoplasmic Reticulum Stress*. Curr Mol Med, 2016. 16(6): p. 533-44.

71.   Xu, M., et al., *Key role of liver sinusoidal endothelial cells in liver fibrosis.* Biosci Trends, 2017. 11(2): p. 163-168.

72.   Horst, A.K., et al., *CEACAM1 in Liver Injury, Metabolic and Immune Regulation.* Int J Mol Sci, 2018. 19(10).

73.   DeAngelis, A.M., et al., *Carcinoembryonic antigen-related cell adhesion molecule 1 - A link between insulin and lipid metabolism.* Diabetes, 2008. 57(9): p. 2296-2303.

74.   Ghosh, S., et al., *Mice with null mutation of Ceacam 1 develop nonalcoholic steatohepatitis.* Hepat Med, 2010. 2010(2): p. 69-78.

75.   Lee, S.J., et al., *Development of nonalcoholic steatohepatitis in insulin-resistant liver-specific S503A carcinoembryonic antigen-related cell adhesion molecule 1 mutant mice.* Gastroenterology, 2008. 135(6): p. 2084-95.

# Chapter 2: Aortic Fibrosis in Insulin-Sensitive Mice with Endothelial Cell Specific

## Deletion of *Ceacam1* Gene

**Introduction**

Atherosclerotic cardiovascular disease is the most common cause of death in the world accounting for an estimate of 31.5% of all global deaths [1]. Individuals with metabolic syndrome are more susceptible to developing atherosclerosis. The metabolic syndrome encompasses a group of abnormalities including visceral obesity, insulin resistance, and a dyslipidemia profile characterized by increased serum triglycerides, decreased HDL cholesterol, and increased small dense LDL cholesterol [41]. The association between metabolic syndrome, dyslipidemia, and increased risk of cardiovascular disease is well documented. However, the role of insulin resistance contributing to each of these abnormalities is still debated.

Carcinoembryonic antigen-related cell adhesion molecule1 (CEACAM1) is a transmembrane glycoprotein that is expressed abundantly in hepatocytes and vascular endothelium. In addition to its function in aiding insulin clearance in the liver, CEACAM1 promotes vascular morphogenesis [2]. Impaired ability to clear insulin causes hyperinsulinemia accompanied with peripheral insulin resistance as a result of downregulation of the insulin receptor [3]. Insulin resistance, manifested by hyperinsulinemia, is the main hallmark of obesity and atherosclerosis [4]. In fact, many studies have demonstrated that insulin resistance can be an independent risk factor of atherosclerosis [42-43].

Many reports have shown that hypercholesterolemia without insulin resistance did not cause atherosclerosis [5]. This current study aimed to investigate the inciting factors that cause atherosclerosis by looking at a possible role of endothelial cell CEACAM1 in contributing to the pathogenesis of this disease. Atherosclerosis involves more than the accumulation of lipids within the artery wall, it is a complex response of the artery to tissue damage and inflammation [6, 7].

Endothelial cell injury is considered the first step in the development of atherosclerosis [8]. Mice with global null deletion of the *Ceacam1* gene develop early atherosclerotic plaque-like lesions in their aortae [9]. These mice suffer hyperinsulinemia resulting from impaired insulin clearance which impairs insulin signaling; this in turn, results in decreased nitric oxide production caused by decreased Akt/eNOS activation resulting in elevated levels of VCAM-1 and pro-inflammatory cytokines [9]. Therefore, global lack of *Ceacam1* drives vascular dysfunction through hyperinsulinemia and ectopic fat accumulation which contributes to the initiation of atherosclerotic plaque-like lesions. Moreover, mice with liver-specific deletion of *Ceacam1* developed atherogenic plaques resulting from systemic insulin resistance and its associated inflammation and fibrosis [10]. Interestingly, siRNA-mediated deletion of *Ceacam1* in bovine endothelial cells showed lower Akt/eNOS activation compared with control. This demonstrated that CEACAM1 could regulate both endothelial cell autonomous and non-autonomous mechanisms involved in vascular morphology and NO production in aortae [9].

The endothelium is responsible for regulating vascular permeability. This function is critical as altered vascular permeability has been reported to aggravate a number of diseases including atherosclerosis [11]. Endothelial cell injury allows more inflammatory molecules into the vessel wall. Endothelial cell damage has been shown to be one of the important pathological events that cause atherosclerosis by a combination of metabolic and inflammatory derangements [6]. Evidence for altered expression of endothelial cell adhesion molecules in inflammation is mounting [12]. During hypoxia and atherosclerosis, CEACAM1 is upregulated to mediate the remodeling of the endothelial barrier function. This suggests an important function of CEACAM1 in maintaining vascular homeostasis [13]. Moreover, reports have shown that overexpression of endothelial-cell specific CEACAM1 in mice improved wrapping of the endothelial barrier by pericytes which allow endothelial cells to differentiate and form vascular branches [14]. This also suggests that CEACAM1 might facilitate heterotypic adhesion between endothelial cells and accessory cells such as pericytes [15]. In addition, there is a prominent evidence for the impact of CEACAM1 in mediating vascular homeostasis in adult blood vessels. Studies on the aorta of $ApoE^{-/-}$ mice showed increased CEACAM1 expression in activated endothelium of atherosclerotic plaques [16]. This demonstrates that CEACAM1 is required for endothelial cell function.

To address the cell-autonomous effect of endothelial CEACAM1 in the pathogenesis of atherosclerosis, the current study examined whether insulin sensitive endothelial-CEACAM1 knockout mice on the $LDLr^{-/-}$ background could be susceptible to atherosclerosis.

**Methods**

*Mice Generation*

Endothelial-cell specific $Cc1^{-/-}$ mouse line was generated by breeding mice having the germline transmission of the loxP-targeted CC1 allele to generate CC1 loxp/loxp mice. CC1 loxp/loxp mice were crossed with transgenic mice having the Cre VE-

Cadherin gene promoter (VECadCre) and propagated on the C57BL6 (BL6) genetic background. These mice were then backcrossed with low density lipoprotein receptor deficient mouse $LDLr^{-/-}$ for more than 6 generations to have four homozygous littermates.

*Mice Genotyping*

Genotyping was done by polymerase chain reaction (PCR) analysis using ear lysates to validate the four littermate groups: $VECad\text{-}Ccl^{+/+}$, $VECad\text{+}Ccl^{+/+}$, $VECad\text{-}Ccl^{fl/fl}$ and $VECad\text{+}Ccl^{fl/fl}$ mice. As seen in Fig. S1, the Flox reaction consisted of a FloxA forward primer and FloxB and FloxC reverse primers. Primer pairs FloxA and FloxB detected the 382bp wild-type allele, while primer pairs FloxA and FloxC detected the 488bp floxed gene. For the Cre reaction, the VECadCre- allele was detected at 550bp, and the VECadCre+ allele was detected at 300bp of the VECadherin promoter and the 550bp of the VECadherin gene. All mice showed the Ldlr mutant band at 350bp using the OMIR33 49 primer forward and the primer reverse pairs OMIR33 50 and OMIR00 92. Nucleotide sequences are listed at the bottom of the illustrations.

*Mice Maintenance*

All animals were housed in a 12-hour dark-light cycle. Starting at 4 months of age, male mice were fed high cholesterol diet (HC) *ad libitum* (Harlan Teklad, TD.88137, Harlan, Haslett, MI) adjusted calories diet (42% from fat), for 2 months; or starting at 6 months of age, male mice were fed high cholesterol diet for 3 month or 5 months. Body weight was assessed weekly. All procedures and animal experiments were approved by the Institutional Animal Care and Utilization Committee at Ohio University.

*Insulin and Glucose Tolerance Tests*

Mice were fasted 7 hours before being subjected to an intraperitoneal injection of insulin (0.75 U/kg BW, Novo Nordisk, Princeton, NJ) (for insulin tolerance) or glucose (1.5 g/kg BW of 50% dextrose solution, Dextrose Injection, USP).

*Tissue and Plasma Biochemistry*

Mice were fasted overnight, and retro-orbital blood was drawn the following morning to assess steady-state levels of plasma insulin (80-INSMSU-E01 ELISA kit; ALPCO, Salem, NH, USA), and C-peptide (80-CPTMS-E01 ELISA kit; ALPCO), non-esterified fatty acids (NEFA-C enzymatic colorimetric assay; Wako Diagnostics, Richmond, VA, USA) and triacylglycerol (Pointe Scientific Triglyceride, Canton, MI, USA). Hepatic triacylglycerol was measured, as previously described [94]. Plasma and hepatic free, total, LDL-VLDL, and HDL cholesterol levels were measured using (Cholesterol assay kit, ab65390, Abcam, Cambridge, MA, USA). Plasma VLDL was calculated by dividing the plasma TG values by 5. Plasma LDL was measured using a Mouse LDL-Cholesterol kit (79980, Crystal chem, Elk Grove Village, IL, USA). Plasma and aortic nitric oxide levels were assessed using a Nitrate/Nitrite Fluorometric Assay Kit (780051, Cayman Chemical, Ann Arbor, MI, USA). Plasma endothelin-1 was measured using an Endothlein-1 ELISA kit (ab133030, Abcam, Cambridge, MA, USA). Plasma NAD/NADH was measured using a Total NAD and NADH colorimetric Assay Kit (ab186032, Abcam, Cambridge, MA, USA), and plasma Glutathione (GSH) levels were assayed using a Glutathione detection assay kit (ab65322, Abcam, Cambridge, MA, USA). Plasma 8-isoprostane was assessed using an 8-isoprostane ELISA kit (ab175819, Abcam, Cambridge, MA, USA). Plasma TNFα was evaluated using a Mouse TNF alpha

SimpleStep ELISA kit (ab208348, Abcam, Cambridge, MA, USA). Mouse plasma

ApoB100 (MBS2502404) and ApoB48 (MBS744267) were measured using

MyBiosource ELISA kits (CA, USA). Plasma prostaglandin E2 was measured using

(prostaglandin E2 ELISA kit, ab133021, Abcam, Cambridge, MA, USA). Plasma PCSK9

was measured using (mouse PCSK9 ELISA kit, ab215538, Abcam, Cambridge, MA,

USA). Plasma IL-6 was measured using (Interleukin-6 ELISA Kit, ab222503). Plasma

Alanine Transaminase (ALT) (ab105134) and Aspartate Aminotransferase (AST)

(ab105135) colorimetric assays kits were measured following the Abcam manufacturer's

protocol.  Plasma PDGF-B was assayed using (ELISA Kit, MBB00; R&D System,

Minneapolis, MN, USA).

*HMG-CoA Reductase Activity Assay*

Mice were fasted overnight, and livers were collected the next day. Livers were

homogenized following manufacturer's instructions (HMG-CoA Reductase Activity

Colorimetric Assay Kit, ab204701, Abcam, Cambridge, MA, USA).

*Aortic Root Sectioning and Plaque Analysis*

Hearts were perfused through the left ventricle with 1x phosphate buffered saline

(PBS) followed by 4% paraformaldehyde (PFA). Hearts were cut in a plane parallel to

the atria and embedded in optimal cutting temperature compound (O.C.T compound,

Tissue-Tek, 4583. CA, USA) followed by sectioning using a microtome-cryostat (10µm

each section). For H&E staining, OCT embedded slides were hydrated in deionized

water. Slides were placed in Hematoxylin for 2 min, followed by rinsing in deionized

water (three times). Slides were then placed in 95% ethanol for 1 min followed by Eosin

Y for 1 min (twice). Slides were dehydrated sequentially in 95% ethanol, and 100% ethanol for 1 min (three times). Slides were cleared with xylene for 1 min (three times) and mounted. For Oil red O staining, OCT embedded aortic root sections were fixed in formalin for 10 min, then hydrated in distilled water (four dips), followed by rinsing with 60% isopropanol. Then, slides were stained with freshly prepared oil red o working solution for 15 min. Slides were rinsed with 60% isopropanol, then placed in alum hematoxylin (four dips). Slides were then rinsed with distilled water and mounted. Image J software was used to quantify positive lipid-stained areas. Sections for Gomori-trichrome staining (87020; Thermo Scientific) were deparaffinized at 60°C and hydrated in deionized water. Sections were then stained with Bouin's Fluid for 45 min at 56°C, followed by rinsing in deionized water. Slides were placed in Working Wright's Iron Hematoxylin for 10 min followed by Trichrome Stain for 15 min at room temperature. Slides were dehydrated sequentially in 1% acetic acid solution for 1 min, 95% ethanol for 1 min, and 100% ethanol for 1 min (twice). Sections were cleared in xylene solution for 1 min (three times) and mounted. Immunohistochemistry on OCT embedded aortic roots sections was done with CD68 antibody (1:300; catalog #MCA1957GA, Bio-Rad, CA, USA) for 3 hours at room temperature prior to incubation with secondary antibody for 1 hour (biotinylated goat anti-rat antibody, catalog #BA-9401, Vector laboratories, CA, USA). Images were taken at 4× using an Olympus SZX7-TR30 microscope and quantified with Image J software.

*En Face Oil Red O Staining*

Aortae were isolated starting from the aortic arch down to the femoral arteries and fixed in 10% formalin for 24 hours. Aortae were cleaned from fat and surrounding tissues under a dissection microscope. Cleaned aortae were washed with running water for 10 minutes, then rinsed with 60% isopropanol. Aortae were stained with oil red O working solution for 15 minutes, followed by rinsing with 60% isopropanol and then with water. Aortae were cut longitudinally and mounted to slide glass with vessel lumen down, covered with a cover slip, then scanned. The total surface ORO-positive area was calculated using ImageJ software.

*Evan's Blue Staining*

Evan's blue dye (50 mg/kg) in saline was injected through jugular vein of the mice using 26G needle and allowed to circulate for 30-45 minutes. After incubation, the dye remaining in the vascular lumen, which did not pass into the aortic wall, was washed out by injecting cold 20 ml of phosphate-buffered saline (PBS) into the left ventricle. The aorta was removed, cleaned from surrounding fat tissue and fixed in 4% Paraformaldehyde (PFA) at room temperature for 1 hour. After fixation, the remaining PFA was removed by washing the aorta with PBS for $3 \times 5$ minutes, then cut it open. Sub-endothelial Evan's Blue deposition was quantified as an indicator of basal aortic permeability using ImageJ software.

*Intravital Microscopy of Leukocyte Adhesion in Carotid Artery*

Mice were sedated with ketamine and xylazine (100/10 mg/kg) and fixed on a 15-cm cell-culture lid in a supine position. The right jugular vein and left carotid artery were exposed through a middle incision followed by injection of 100 µL of 0.5 mg/mL rhodamine 6G (R4127; Sigma-Aldrich) through the jugular vein puncture to label cells having mitochondria, including leukocytes. The carotid artery was carefully isolated from the surrounding tissue, and one piece of small, U-shaped, black plastic was placed under the vessel to block background fluorescence [48, 49]. The carotid artery (~4-5 mm length) was observed in real time using an intravital microscope (Leica DM6 FS), and video images were captured with a 14-bit RetigaR1 charge-coupled device color digital camera (Teledyne QImaging, Surrey, Canada) and STP7-S-STDT Streampix7 software (Norpix, Montreal, Canada). Video images were analyzed offline for leukocyte adhesion. Cells that adhered to the vessel wall without rolling or moving for at least 3 seconds were counted over the vessel observed. Total numbers were used for statistical analysis.

*Western Blot Analysis*

Aortae or livers or heart endothelial cells were lysed and proteins analyzed by SDS-PAGE followed by immunoprobing with polyclonal antibodies (Cell signaling, Danvers, MA) against: phospho-Akt (Ser 473), Akt, phospho-p44/42 MAPK (Thr 202/Tyr204), p44/42 MAPK, phospho-eNOS (Ser 1177), eNOS, phospho-Smad2Ser465/467, Smad2, phospho-Smad3Ser423/425, Smad3, phospho-Stat3 (Y705), Stat3, phospho-NF-ĶB (S536), NF-ĶB, phospho-PKCζ (phosphothreonine-Thr 410/403), PKCζ, phospho-VEGFR2 (Y1175), and VEGF-R2. Custom-made rabbit polyclonal antibody (Ab 3759) were used against mouse CEACAM1 extracellular domain and phospho-CEACAM1 (α-pCC1) (Bethyl Laboratories, Montgomery, TX). Blots were incubated with horseradish peroxidase-conjugated donkey anti-rabbit IgG antibody (GE Healthcare Life Sciences, Amersham, Marlborough, MA) and proteins were visualized using ECL (Amersham). Polyclonal antibodies against SHP2, and Shc (Cell signaling) were used in co-immunoprecipitation experiments. These membranes were incubated with light chain specific horseradish peroxidase-conjugated IgG monoclonal mouse anti-rabbit (Cat# 211-032- 171, Jackson Immuno-Research laboratories) to prevent detection of the antibody heavy chain.

*Real-Time Quantitative RT-PCR*

Total RNA was isolated from the aortae with RNeasy fibrous tissue kit (Cat #74704) and from livers with NucleoSpin RNA Kit (740955.50, Macherey-Nagel, Bethlehem, PA). cDNA was synthesized by iScript cDNA Synthesis Kit (BIO-RAD), using 1 μg of total RNA and oligodT primers. cDNA was evaluated with quantitative RT-PCR (qRT-PCR; StepOne Plus, Applied Biosystems), and mRNA was normalized to 18S.

*Statistical Analysis*

Data were analyzed by one-way analysis of variance (ANOVA) with Tukey's for multiple comparisons using GraphPad Prism 7 software. $P<0.05$ was considered statistically significant.

**Results**

*Insulin sensitivity and normal cholesterol homeostasis in VECadCre+Ccl$^{fl/fl}$ mice propagated on C57BL6 background*

qRT-PCR analysis demonstrated deletion of *Ceacam1* in endothelial cells from the hearts and livers of *VECadCre+Ccl$^{fl/fl}$* mice (Table 1). In contrast, *Ceacam1* mRNA was intact in their bone marrow macrophages, hepatocytes, and hepatic stellate cells (HSC)

(Table 1).

Compared to control littermates, *VECadCre+Ccl*$^{fl/fl}$ nulls exhibited normal body weight and food intake, leading to intact lean and fat mass up to 12 months of age (Fig. 1A). Visceral adipose mass, and plasma NEFA and adiponectin levels were normal (as shown at 8-9 months of age-Table 2). Null mice also displayed normal steady-state insulin relating to intact insulin secretion (plasma C-peptide) and clearance (steady-state C-peptide/insulin molar ratio). In support of insulin sensitivity, null mice displayed fed normoglycemia (Table 2) and remained tolerant to exogenous insulin and glucose until 12 months (Fig. 1B) and 16 months of age (not shown). Moreover, hepatic and plasma triacylglycerol levels were normal (Table 2). Similarly, plasma cholesterol levels (total, free, VLDL, LDL and HDL) were all normal in *VECadCre+Ccl*$^{fl/fl}$ nulls by comparison to all three control groups (Table 2).

*VECadCre+Ccl*$^{fl/fl}$ *mice display normal histology in aortae*

En-face analysis of aortae revealed no fat deposition in the aorta of *VECadCre+Ccl*$^{fl/fl}$ nulls compared with the Flox control (Fig. 2A). Oil red-O staining of aortic root sections showed absence of steatosis in *VECadCre+Ccl*$^{fl/fl}$ propagated on C57BL6 genetic background as compared to control mice (Fig. 2B). Similarly, Trichrome staining failed to detect fibrosis in the aortae of *VECadCre+Ccl*$^{fl/fl}$ nulls (Fig. 2B).

*Intact insulin sensitivity in the presence of hypercholesterolemia in Ldlr*$^{-/-}$. *VECadCre+Ccl*$^{fl/fl}$ *mice propagated on C57BL6.Ldlr*$^{-/-}$ *background*

Failure of *VECadCre+Ccl*$^{fl/fl}$ nulls propagated on C57BL6 background to develop histological abnormalities could possibly stem from the absence of insulin resistance and/or hypercholesterolemia. To test this hypothesis, we propagated these mice on the hypercholesterolemic C57BL6.*Ldlr*$^{-/-}$ background and fed them at 6 months of age a high-cholesterol (HC) atherogenic diet for 3 months. *Ldlr*$^{-/-}$. *VECadCre+Ccl*$^{fl/fl}$ nulls displayed a comparable diet- and age-related increase in body weight as their littermate controls in response to HC intake (Fig. 3A). This was supported by normal body weight and visceral adipose mass in the nulls relative to controls at 9 months of age (Table 3). Steady-state plasma insulin levels were normal in association with intact insulin secretion (plasma C-peptide and fasting normoglycemia) and clearance (steady-state C-peptide/insulin molar ratio) (Table 3). Together with normal tolerance to exogenous insulin and glucose (Fig. 3B and 3C, respectively), normo-insulinemia and fed normo-glycemia provided an *in vivo* demonstration of insulin sensitivity in *Ldlr*$^{-/-}$ *VECadCre+Ccl*$^{fl/fl}$ mice. Of note, prolonged HC feeding for 5 months did not alter insulin sensitivity in null relative to controls (Fig. S2).

Consistent with normal visceral adiposity, null mice exhibited intact plasma NEFA and triacylglycerol levels in addition to normal hepatic triacylglycerol levels at 9 months of age (Table 3). In contrast, plasma LDL cholesterol (LDL-C) and total cholesterol levels were significantly elevated in *Ldlr*$^{-/-}$. *VECadCre+Ccl*$^{fl/fl}$ compared to controls (Table 3). This did not derive from any change in cholesterol synthesis, as supported by normal activity of hepatic HMG-CoA reductase in nulls compared to controls (Table 3) [18]. Instead, it likely derived from reduced LDL clearance as suggested by the higher plasma ApoB, in particular ApoB100, and proprotein convertase subtilisin/kexin type 9 (PCSK9) levels (Table 3), leading to reduction in LDL-C transport in null mice (39). Consistently, the mRNA levels of hepatic Pcsk9 were ~2-to-4–fold higher and of hepatic LDL receptor-related protein 1 (Lrp1) that is involved in hepatocytic clearance of chylomicron remnants were 2-fold lower in null mice. Together, this demonstrates that *Ldlr⁻ᐟ⁻.VECadCre+Ccl¹ᶠˡ/ᶠˡ* developed an atherogenic dyslipidemic profile when propagated on the C57BL6.*Ldlr⁻ᐟ⁻* background [19, 20].

*Ldlr⁻ᐟ⁻. VECadCre+Ccl¹ᶠˡ/ᶠˡ mice did not display an increase in lipid accumulation in aortae*

En-face analysis of aortae revealed no difference in the fat deposition along the whole aorta between *Ldlr⁻ᐟ⁻. VECadCre+Ccl¹ᶠˡ/ᶠˡ* and their aged-matched littermate controls even after 5 months of atherogenic HC diet intake (Fig. 4A and accompanying graph) and despite increased total plasma cholesterol and ~2-fold increase in plasma LDL-C/VLDL-C levels (Fig. 4B). Similarly, Oil red-O staining of the aortic root cross-sections revealed no significant change in fat deposition in the aortae of HC-fed *Ldlr⁻ᐟ⁻. VECadCre+Ccl¹ᶠˡ/ᶠˡ* mice (Fig. 4C).

*Elevated pro-inflammatory state in Ldlr⁻ᐟ⁻. VECadCre+Ccl¹ᶠˡ/ᶠˡ aortae*

Inflammation is a key factor in the development of pro-fibrotic diseases such as atherosclerosis [21, 22]. Consistently, deleting Ceacam1 from endothelial cells induced the macrophage pool (mRNA of F4/80) (Table S2) and its activation (CD68 immunohistochemical analysis-Fig. 5A) in *Ldlr⁻ᐟ⁻. VECadCre+Ccl¹ᶠˡ/ᶠˡ* aortae compared to all three controls. qRT-PCR analysis revealed an increase in the mRNA levels of pro-inflammatory CD4+T and CD8+T cells, but not the anti-inflammatory Treg pools (Foxp3) in *Ldlr⁻ᐟ⁻. VECadCre+Ccl¹ᶠˡ/ᶠˡ* aortae (Table S2). Normal mRNA levels of IL-4 and IL-13 (Table S2), points to CD4$^+$Th1 response in null aortae.

Activated macrophages and increased inflammatory response was supported by the higher production of pro-inflammatory cytokines (IL-1β; IL-6; TNFα) (Table S2) and their release into the plasma (Fig. 5B). Mechanistically, this could stem from the activation (phosphorylation) of their transcriptional up regulator (NF-κB) in aortae (Fig.5C) and in isolated endothelial cells (Fig. 6C). We have demonstrated that upon its phosphorylation by insulin and epidermal growth factor receptors [38-39], CEACAM1 binds to and sequesters Shc to reduce its coupling to growth factor receptors and downregulate the ras/MAPK downstream signaling pathways. This would also lead to NF-kB inactivation. Similarly, treatment of primary endothelial cells isolated from the hearts of 2-month-old *Ldlr*$^{-/-}$ mice with VEGF-A (40ng/ml) for 5 minutes detected a stronger level of VEGFR2 in the immunopellet of Shc in cells derived from *VECadCre+Ccl*$^{fl/fl}$ mice than their control counterparts (Fig. 6A). This led to a higher phosphorylation of MAPK (Fig. 6B) and NF-kB (Fig. 6C) in null than control endothelial cells.

IL-6 can activate the STAT3 (signal transducer and activator of transcription 3) inflammatory pathway [23]. Accordingly, *Ldlr*$^{-/-}$. *VECadCre+Ccl*$^{fl/fl}$ aortae exhibited enhanced STAT3 phosphorylation (activation) compared with controls (Fig. 5C). Together with NF-κB activation, this induced the mRNA levels of the monocyte chemoattractant protein-1 (Mcp-1), Toll-like receptors 2/4 (Tlr-2/4) and the Cd11b+ macrophage pool [40] (Table S2). The data demonstrate that null deletion of *Ceacam1* in endothelial cells causes a cell-autonomous positive effect on NF-kB and Stat3 activation and its downstream transcriptional targets to alter the inflammatory microenvironment in *Ldlr*$^{-/-}$. *VECadCre+Ccl*$^{fl/fl}$ aortae.

*Increased endothelial cell permeability in Ldlr$^{-/-}$. VECadCre+Ccl$^{fl/fl}$ mice*

Endothelial CEACAM1 regulates the expression of factors critical to the formation of endothelial barrier [16] to prevent vascular permeability [13]. Accordingly, Evans blue injection in jugular vein revealed ~3-4–fold higher incorporation on the surface of *Ldlr$^{-/-}$. VECadCre+Ccl$^{fl/fl}$* aortae than controls (Fig. 7A), indicating more vascular permeability in the nulls relative to their controls. This was supported by ~2-to-3–fold decrease in the mRNA levels of genes involved in the formation of tight junctions (Zo-1, Claudin1, Claudin2, Occludin) and in maintaining vascular integrity (VE-Cadherin and b-catenin, VEGF-A and its receptor VEGFR-2, VEGFR1 and angiopoietins (Ang-1/2) in *Ldlr$^{-/-}$. VECadCre+Ccl$^{fl/fl}$* aortae compared to controls (Table S3).  Western blot analysis confirmed reduction of VEGFR2 in the lysates of *Ldlr$^{-/-}$. VECadCre+Ccl$^{fl/fl}$* aortae relative to controls (Fig. 7B). At the cellular level, activation of PKCζ/NF-kB pathways (Fig. 5C) by elevated TNFα could contribute to increased endothelial cell permeability in the aortae of *Ldlr$^{-/-}$. VECadCre+Ccl$^{fl/fl}$* versus control mice.

Consistent with increased inflammation and vascular permeability, deleting *Ceacam1* from endothelial cells induced leukocyte adhesion to the vessel wall of the nulls, as indicated by intravital microscopy of the carotid artery (Fig. 7C). Additionally, this is supported by the significant increase in the mRNA levels of the vascular cell adhesion molecule (VCAM-1) that mediates leukocyte-endothelial adhesion (Table S2), as we expected from our previous observations on increased VCAM-1 protein levels in bovine aortic endothelial cells with SiRNA-mediated downregulation of Ceacam1 [9].

*Increased lipid peroxidation and oxidative stress in Ldlr$^{-/-}$. VECadCre+Ccl$^{fl/fl}$ mice.*

Oxidative stress plays a central role in cardiovascular disorders [21, 24]. qRT-PCR analysis of aorta showed increased aortic mRNA levels of NOX4 as well as higher levels of GP91 in *Ldlr$^{-/-}$. VECadCre+Cc1$^{fl/fl}$* mice fed 3 months of atherogenic diet (Table S3). Additionally, 3 months of HC intake, null mice exhibited an increase in plasma NAD/NADH and 8-isoprostane levels (Fig. 8A.a and 8A.b, respectively) with a reciprocal decrease in plasma nitric oxide (NO) levels in nulls versus control mice (Fig. 8A.c). Moreover, qRT-PCR analysis revealed a significant reduction in Niemann-Pick type C1 protein (NPC-1) in *Ldlr$^{-/-}$. VECadCre+Cc1$^{fl/fl}$* aortae (Table S3) in association with a marked reduction in plasma GSH levels (Fig. 8A.d), which could contribute to the robust response to the cytotoxic effects of TNFα.

Inflammation and oxidative stress mediate endothelial injury resulting from low NO bioavailability [25]. Consistently, *Ldlr$^{-/-}$. VECadCre+Cc1$^{fl/fl}$* mice exhibited lower aortic levels of NO (Fig. 8B) following 3 months of HC intake. Western analysis of lysates of primary endothelial cells treated with VEGF-A for 5 minutes revealed increased binding of SHP2 to VEGFR2 (Fig. 9B) in the absence of SHP2 sequestration by CEACAM1 (Fig. 9A), leading to its reduced phosphorylation in *Ldlr$^{-/-}$. VECadCre+Cc1$^{fl/fl}$* mice (Fig. 9B). This led to inactivation of Akt/eNOS downstream signaling pathway (Fig. 9C-D), as we have previously shown [9]. Consistently, VEGF activation failed to induce NO production and release in the medium of endothelial cells derived from *Ldlr$^{-/-}$. VECadCre+Cc1$^{fl/fl}$* mice as it did in control cells (Fig. 9E).

*Increased fibrosis in the aortic root of Ldlr$^{-/-}$. VECadCre+Cc1$^{fl/fl}$ mice*

Gomori trichrome staining indicates sub-endothelial accumulation of fibrotic content in the aortic root of *Ldlr*$^{-/-}$. *VECadCre+Ccl1*$^{fl/fl}$ mice compared with their age-matched littermate controls after 3 months (not shown) and 4 months of HC feeding (Fig. 10A and accompanying graph). Moreover, qRT-PCR analysis revealed a 2-to-5–fold increase in aortic mRNA levels of fibrosis markers: fibronectin, Ctgf, α-Sma, collagen6α3 and Tgfb in *Ldlr*$^{-/-}$. *VECadCre+Ccl1*$^{fl/fl}$ relative to controls after 3 months of HC feeding (Table S3). Consistent with the ~3-fold decrease in the mRNA level of Smad7, an inhibitor of the TGFb–Smad2/3 canonical pathway, this pro-fibrogenic pathway was more highly activated (phosphorylated) in *Ldlr*$^{-/-}$. *VECadCre+Ccl1*$^{fl/fl}$ relative to controls (Fig. 10B).

Elevated fibrogenesis in *Ldlr*$^{-/-}$. *VECadCre+Ccl1*$^{fl/fl}$ could be mediated by increased NF-kB-mediated transcription of endothelin-1 (ET-1) and their release from their endothelial cells (Fig. 6D). This could contribute to increased mRNA of aortic ET1 and its receptor-A (Etar) (Table S3) and in the plasma levels of ET1 in *Ldlr*$^{-/-}$. *VECadCre+Ccl1*$^{fl/fl}$ mice compared to controls (Fig. 6E). Increased plasma levels of PGE2 (Fig. 6E) could also contribute to the ~2-fold increase in the plasma levels of ET-1 in *Ldlr*$^{-/-}$. *VECadCre+Ccl1*$^{fl/fl}$ mice relative to the control littermates. In addition to ET-1, NF-kB activation stimulates the transcription of PDGF-B to contribute to its increased plasma levels (Fig. 6E) and synergize with ET1 to mediate fibrogenesis.

**Discussion**

Outcome studies have shown that lowering plasma cholesterol levels was not effective in stopping the progression of atherosclerosis in patients with metabolic diseases [26]. This emphasizes the central role of insulin resistance in the development of atherosclerosis [43]. Clarifying the pathogenic link between endothelial cell injury, metabolic derangements, and atherosclerosis has been challenging [27]. This is partially due to the lack of mouse models that mimic the aspects of the disease. Current mouse models of atherosclerosis depend on extensive hypercholesterolemia bestowed by either $Ldlr^{-/-}$ or $ApoE^{-/-}$ background and metabolic complications such as obesity and insulin resistance to induce atherosclerosis [28, 29]. This complicates the investigation of the development of the disease and can override any effects that otherwise could be contributing to atherosclerosis. Therefore, the atherogenic mouse model of endothelial cell specific *Ceacam1* deletion provides hypercholesterolemia with whole-body insulin sensitivity, hence can be used to pinpoint the role of insulin resistance in the pathogenesis of atherosclerosis in the absence of systemic risk factors. As well as this insulin sensitive mouse model can target the inflammatory and fibrotic processes to better identify novel means of treating this vascular disease.

VEGF signaling prevents endothelial injury that can initiate atherogenesis [30]. Moreover, injury to the vascular endothelium provokes an inflammatory response causing the release of cell surface adhesion molecules. This changes the endothelial cell morphology resulting in increased permeability of lipids and fluids to the intimal endothelium [21]. Our conditional knockout mice revealed decreased expression of VEGF-R2 as well as increased vascular permeability as evident in the Evans blue stain of the whole aorta. This vascular endothelium injury resulted in a proinflammatory state as demonstrated by increased adhesion of leukocytes to the vascular endothelium. In addition, we observed aortic increase of inflammatory, vasoconstrictor, and oxidative stress factors.

Most importantly, after 3 months of high cholesterol diet, our endothelial cell specific CEACAM1 knockout mice demonstrated significantly higher levels of plasma TNF-$\alpha$, IL-6, GSH, and NAD/NADH. This revealed oxidative stress, lipid peroxidation, and inflammation in the VECad+Cc1$^{fl/fl}$ mice compared to controls. This indeed suggests that endothelial CEACAM1 plays an important role in vascular homeostasis and endothelial barrier regulation.

Several reports have concluded that plaque composition denotes plaque rupture [31]. Thus, the key characteristics of a vulnerable plaque include the presence of a thin fibrous cap (<65µm), enlarged necrotic core (occupies more than 30% of total plaque), the occurrence of hemorrhage, and substantial infiltration of inflammatory cells [32]. A vulnerable necrotic core is defined by the buildup of free cholesterol and lack of supporting collagen [31]. We did not observe alternations in the plasma free cholesterol levels in our *VECad+Cc1$^{fl/fl}$* mice and their littermate controls. Moreover, based on the trichrome staining of aortic rings, our VECad+Cc1$^{fl/fl}$ mice developed fibrosis compared with controls without significant changes to lipid deposition in their aortic roots or whole aorta. This indicates increased sub-endothelial accumulation of fibrotic content which perhaps is limiting vulnerable plaque formation.

Additionally, our VECad+Cc1$^{fl/fl}$ mice showed higher plasma LDL and total cholesterol levels compared with littermate controls which we expect is caused by reduced plasma LDL clearance [33]. PCSK9 contributes to cholesterol homeostasis by inhibiting the degradation of hepatic lipoprotein receptors [34]. Our VECad+Cc1$^{fl/fl}$ mice showed higher plasma PCSK9 levels as well as elevated hepatic PCSK9 expression compared with littermate controls. Hence, expression of PCSK9 promotes the degradation of hepatic lipoprotein uptake receptors such as LRP1 [35] as we have observed.

The current study established the presence of compromised vasodilation and development of fibrosis in the aortic roots of the endothelial cell specific CEACAM1 knockout mice on the *Ldlr*⁻/⁻ background compared to controls. We suggest that this fibrotic phenotype shed from increased endothelin-1 and PDGF-B levels. Together, results of this study assigned insulin resistance a critical role in driving overt atherosclerosis [36] [37].

**Figure Legends**

*Figure 1:* Body weight and daily food intake in endothelial cell CEACAM1 knockout mice on the C57Bl6 background. (**A**) Body weight change and food intake were assessed starting from 3 or 5 to 12 months of age, respectively, in male mice ($n$=5-6 for each genotype and age group). Values are expressed as mean $\pm$ SEM; (*VECadCre–Ccl*$^{+/+}$ (green), *VECadCre+Ccl*$^{+/+}$ (blue), *VECadCre–Ccl*$^{fl/fl}$ (purple) and null *VECadCre+Ccl*$^{fl/fl}$ (red). Analysis of insulin sensitivity. 12-month-old male mice ($n\geq$7-8/genotype/age group) were injected intraperitoneally with insulin or glucose to assess (**B**) insulin and glucose tolerance. Values were expressed as mean±SEM; *VECad–Ccl*$^{+/+}$ (Wild-type controls), *VECad+Ccl*$^{+/+}$ (Cre controls), *VECad–Ccl*$^{fl/fl}$ (Flox controls) and *VECad+Ccl*$^{fl/fl}$ (null mice).

*Figure 2:* En-face and aortic root histology of 9 months old male (**A**) En-face of whole aortae of *a.* VECad-Ccl$^{fl/fl}$ and *b.* VECad+Ccl$^{fl/fl}$ mice. (**B**) Aortic root staining of *a.* VECad-Ccl$^{+/+,}$ *b.* VECad+Ccl$^{+/+}$, *c.* VECad-Ccl$^{fl/fl}$ and *d.* VECad+Ccl$^{fl/fl}$ mice (*a*) Oil red O staining of aortic roots. (*b*) CD68 staining of aortic roots. (*c*) Trichrome staining of aortic roots. Both accompanied with quantification graphs calculated as area pixel$^2$ using ImageJ.

*Figure 3:* Analysis of insulin sensitivity and body weight in endothelial cell CEACAM1 knockout mice propagated on the Ldlr background. 6 months old male VECad+Ccl$^{fl/fl}$ mice and their controls (n>5 per group) were fed high cholesterol diet for 3 months (**A**) Body weight was assessed weekly over a 3-month period of high cholesterol intake. Mice were subjected to an intraperitoneal injection of (**B**) insulin (0.75 U/kg BW),

(**C**) glucose (1.5 g/kg BW) to evaluate blood glucose levels at 0-180 min post-injection and 1-120 respectively.

*Figure 4:* Morphologic analysis of aortic lesions. 6 months old male *a.* VECad-Ccl$^{+/+,}$ *b.* VECad+Ccl$^{+/+}$, *c.* VECad-Ccl$^{fl/fl}$ and *d.* VECad+Ccl$^{fl/fl}$ mice after 5 months of high cholesterol diet were assessed for (**A**) En-face analysis of aortic surface lesions. (**B**) Plasma cholesterol levels. Values are expressed as mean ± SEM. *$P<0.05$ vs. VECad-Ccl$^{+/+,}$ VECad+Ccl$^{+/+}$, and VECad-Ccl$^{fl/fl}$. (**C**) Oil red O staining of aortic roots after 3 months of high cholesterol diet were assessed. Both accompanied with quantification graphs calculated as area pixel$^2$ using ImageJ.

*Figure 5:* Vascular inflammation and leukocyte adhesion. (**A**) IHC analysis of CD68 in aortic roots of 6 months old male *a.* VECad-Ccl$^{+/+,}$ *b.* VECad+Ccl$^{+/+}$, *c.* VECad-Ccl$^{fl/fl}$ and *d.* VECad+Ccl$^{fl/fl}$ mice after 3 months of high cholesterol feeding, accompanied with quantification of positive stained areas calculated as area pixel$^2$ using imageJ. *$P<0.05$ vs. VECad-Ccl$^{+/+,}$ VECad+Ccl$^{+/+}$, and VECad-Ccl$^{fl/fl}$. (**B**) Retro-orbital venous blood was drawn from overnight fasted *a.* VECad-Ccl$^{+/+,}$ *b.* VECad+Ccl$^{+/+}$, *c.* VECad-Ccl$^{fl/fl}$ and *d.* VECad+Ccl$^{fl/fl}$ mice (n>5 per group). Plasma was analyzed for (**B.***a*) TNFα, (**B.***b*) IL-6. Values are expressed as mean ± SEM. *$P<0.05$ vs. VECad-Ccl$^{+/+,}$ VECad+Ccl$^{+/+}$, and VECad-Ccl$^{fl/fl}$. (**C**) Aortic lysates were analyzed by immunoblotting (Ib) using antibodies against α-phospho-STAT3, α-phospho-NF-κB, and α-phospho-PKCζ followed by probing with α-STAT3, α-NF-κB, and α-PKCζ respectively, for normalization.

*Figure 6:* Insulin/ VEGF signaling in endothelial cells. Primary heart endothelial cells from VECad-Ccl$^{+/+}$, VECad+Ccl$^{+/+}$, VECad-Ccl$^{fl/fl}$ and *VECad+Ccl$^{fl/fl}$* mice were treated with or without VEGF-A (40ng/ml) for 5 minutes. **(A)** Lysates were subjected to co-immunoprecipitation with Shc antibody followed by immunoblotting with antibodies against phospho-CEACAM1 (pCC1) and phospho-VEGFR2 (pVEGFR2). **(B-C)** lysates were subjected to immunoblotting with α-phospho- antibodies against MAPK and NF-κB respectively. **(D)** ET-1 was evaluated in the media of the primary heart endothelial cells following 20 minutes stimulation with VEGF-A (40ng/ml). Values are expressed as mean ± SEM. [a]$P<0.05$ vs. absence (-) of VEGF-A, [b]$P<0.05$ absence (-) of VEGF-A in the controls vs. null, [c]$P<0.05$ presence (+) of VEGF-A in the controls vs. null. **(E)** Retro-orbital venous blood was drawn from overnight fasted mice (n>5 per group). Plasma was analyzed for ET-1, PGE2, and PDGF-B. Values are expressed as mean ± SEM. *$P<0.05$ vs. VECad-Cc1$^{+/+,}$ VECad+Cc1$^{+/+}$, and VECad-Cc1$^{fl/fl}$.

*Figure 7:* Assessing vascular permeability. 9 months old male *a.* VECad-Cc1$^{+/+,}$ *b.* VECad+Cc1$^{+/+}$, *c.* VECad-Cc1$^{fl/fl}$ and *d.* VECad+Cc1$^{fl/fl}$ mice were subjected to Evans blue injection via the jugular vein. **(A)** Images of aortae stained with Evans's blue accompanied by quantification of positive stained areas calculated as area pixel$^2$ using ImageJ, *$P<0.05$ vs. VECad-Cc1$^{+/+,}$ VECad+Cc1$^{+/+}$, and VECad-Cc1$^{fl/fl}$. **(B)** Aortic lysates were analyzed by immunoblotting (Ib) using antibodies against α-VEGF-R2 followed by probing with α-Tubulin for normalization. **(C)** Intravital microscopy of leukocyte adhesion in carotid artery was assessed in *a.* VECad+Cc1$^{+/+}$, *b.* VECad-Cc1$^{fl/fl}$ and *c.* VECad+Cc1$^{fl/fl}$ mice after 5 months of high cholesterol feeding. Cells that adhered to the vessel wall without rolling for at least 3 seconds were counted by using an intravital microscope. Video images were analyzed offline for leukocyte adhesion. Total numbers were used for statistical analysis. *$P<0.05$ vs. VECad+Ccl$^{+/+}$, and VECad-Ccl$^{fl/fl}$.

*Figure 8:* Assessing redox parameters. 6 months old male VECad+Ccl$^{fl/fl}$ mice and their controls were fed a high cholesterol diet for 3 months. Retro-orbital venous blood was drawn from overnight fasted mice (n>5 per group). Plasma was analyzed for (**A.***a*) NAD/NADH, (**A.***b*) 8-Isoprostane, (**A.***c*) nitric oxide levels, and (**A.***d*) GSH. (**B**) Aortae were lysed and NO content was measured. Values are expressed as mean ± SEM. *$P<0.05$ vs. VECad-Ccl$^{+/+,}$ VECad+Ccl$^{+/+}$, and VECad-Ccl$^{fl/fl}$.

*Figure 9:* Insulin/VEGF signaling in endothelial cells. Primary heart endothelial cells from VECad-Ccl$^{+/+}$, VECad+Ccl$^{+/+}$, VECad-Ccl$^{fl/fl}$ and *VECad+Ccl$^{fl/fl}$* mice were treated with or without VEGF-A (40ng/ml) for 5 minutes. (**A**) Lysates were subjected to co-immunoprecipitation with SHP2 antibody followed by immunoblotting with antibodies against phospho-CEACAM1 (pCC1) and CEACAM1 (CC1). (**B**) Lysates were subjected to co-immunoprecipitation with SHP2 antibody followed by immunoblotting with antibodies against phospho-VEGFR2 and VEGFR2. (**C-D**) lysates were subjected to immunoblotting with α-phospho- antibodies against Akt and eNOS respectively. (**E**) NO was evaluated in the media of the primary heart endothelial cells following 20 minutes stimulation with VEGF-A (40ng/ml). Values are expressed as mean ± SEM. $^{a}P<0.05$ vs. absence (-) of VEGF-A, $^{b}P<0.05$ absence (-) of VEGF-A in the controls vs. null, $^{c}P<0.05$ presence (+) of VEGF-A in the controls vs. null.

*Figure 10:* Assessing vascular fibrosis. (**A**) Gomori trichrome staining of aortic roots of 6 months old male *a.* VECad-Ccl$^{+/+,}$ *b.* VECad+Ccl$^{+/+}$, *c.* VECad-Ccl$^{fl/fl}$ and *d.*

VECad+Ccl$^{fl/fl}$ mice after 4 months of high cholesterol feeding, accompanied with quantification of positive areas calculated as area pixel$^2$ using imageJ. *$P<0.05$ vs. VECad-Ccl$^{+/+,}$ VECad+Ccl$^{+/+}$, and VECad-Ccl$^{fl/fl}$. (**B**) Aortic lysates were analyzed by immunoblotting with α-phospho-Smad2 (α-pSmad2), and α-phospho-Smad3 (α-pSmad3) antibodies followed by immuno probing with antibodies against total Smad2, and total Smad3, respectively, for normalization.

*Figure S1:* Mice genotyping using ear lysates. (**A**) Flox reaction, (**B**) VE-Cad Cre, (**C**) LDLr reaction. Nucleotide sequences are listed in the table at the bottom of the agarose gels.

*Figure S2:* Analysis of insulin sensitivity. (**A**) 6 months old male VECad+Ccl$^{fl/fl}$ mice and their controls (n>5 per group) were fed high cholesterol diet for 5 months and then were subjected to an intraperitoneal injection of insulin (0.75 U/kg BW) to evaluate blood glucose levels at 0-180 min post-injection. Insulin tolerance was measured as percentage of basal blood glucose level.

**References**

1.	DeAngelis, A.M., et al., *Carcinoembryonic antigen-related cell adhesion molecule 1 - A link between insulin and lipid metabolism.* Diabetes, 2008. 57(9): p. 2296-2303.

2.	Russo, L., et al., *Liver-specific rescuing of CEACAM1 reverses endothelial and cardiovascular abnormalities in male mice with null deletion of Ceacam1 gene.* Mol Metab, 2018. 9: p. 98-113.

3.	Najjar, S.M., et al., *Ceacam1 deletion causes vascular alterations in large vessels.* Am J Physiol Endocrinol Metab, 2013. 305(4): p. E519-29.

4.	Benjamin, E.J., et al., *Heart Disease and Stroke Statistics-2017 Update: A Report From the American Heart Association.* Circulation, 2017. 135(10): p. e146-e603.

5.	Najjar, S.M., *Regulation of insulin action by CEACAM1.* Trends Endocrinol Metab, 2002. 13(6): p. 240-5.

6.	Russo, L., et al., *Liver-specific reconstitution of CEACAM1 reverses the metabolic abnormalities caused by its global deletion in male mice.* Diabetologia, 2017. 60(12): p. 2463-2474.

7.	Di Pino, A. and R.A. DeFronzo, *Insulin Resistance and Atherosclerosis: Implications for Insulin-Sensitizing Agents.* Endocr Rev, 2019. 40(6): p. 1447-1467.

8.	Heinrich, G., et al., *Loss of Hepatic CEACAM1: A Unifying Mechanism Linking Insulin Resistance to Obesity and Non-Alcoholic Fatty Liver Disease.* Front Endocrinol (Lausanne), 2017. 8: p. 8.

9.      Tsuchiya, K., et al., *FoxOs integrate pleiotropic actions of insulin in vascular endothelium to protect mice from atherosclerosis.* Cell Metab, 2012. 15(3): p. 372-81.

10.     Vita, J.A., et al., *Coronary vasomotor response to acetylcholine relates to risk factors for coronary artery disease.* Circulation, 1990. 81(2): p. 491-7.

11.     Varghese, J.F., R. Patel, and U.C.S. Yadav, *Novel insights in the metabolic syndrome-induced oxidative stress and inflammation-mediated atherosclerosis.* Curr Cardiol Rev, 2017.

12.     Khalil, M.F., W.D. Wagner, and I.J. Goldberg, *Molecular interactions leading to lipoprotein retention and the initiation of atherosclerosis.* Arterioscler Thromb Vasc Biol, 2004. 24(12): p. 2211-8.

13.     Frank, P.G. and M.P. Lisanti, *ICAM-1: role in inflammation and in the regulation of vascular permeability.* Am J Physiol Heart Circ Physiol, 2008. 295(3): p. H926-H927.

14.     Reglero-Real, N., et al., *Endothelial Cell Junctional Adhesion Molecules: Role and Regulation of Expression in Inflammation.* Arterioscler Thromb Vasc Biol, 2016. 36(10): p. 2048-2057.

15.     Rueckschloss, U., S. Kuerten, and S. Ergun, *The role of CEA-related cell adhesion molecule-1 (CEACAM1) in vascular homeostasis.* Histochem Cell Biol, 2016. 146(6): p. 657-671.

16.     Gerstel, D., et al., *CEACAM1 creates a pro-angiogenic tumor microenvironment that supports tumor vessel maturation.* Oncogene, 2011. 30(41): p. 4275-4288.

17.     Wagener, C. and S. Ergun, *Angiogenic properties of the carcinoembryonic antigen-related cell adhesion molecule 1.* Exp Cell Res, 2000. 261(1): p. 19-24.

18.     Ghavampour, S., et al., *Endothelial barrier function is differentially regulated by CEACAM1-mediated signaling.* FASEB J, 2018. 32(10): p. 5612-5625.

19.     Russo, L., et al., *Role for hepatic CEACAM1 in regulating fatty acid metabolism along the adipocyte-hepatocyte axis.* J Lipid Res, 2016. 57(12): p. 2163-2175.

20.     Li, Y., et al., *A novel role for CRTC2 in hepatic cholesterol synthesis through SREBP-2.* Hepatology, 2017. 66(2): p. 481-497.

21.     Marchio, P., et al., *Targeting Early Atherosclerosis: A Focus on Oxidative Stress and Inflammation.* Oxid Med Cell Longev, 2019. 2019: p. 8563845.

22.     Li, B., et al., *Inflammation: A Novel Therapeutic Target/Direction in Atherosclerosis.* Curr Pharm Des, 2017. 23(8): p. 1216-1227.

23.     Chen, Q., et al., *Targeted inhibition of STAT3 as a potential treatment strategy for atherosclerosis.* Theranostics, 2019. 9(22): p. 6424-6442.

24.     Ueda, Y., et al., *Reduction of 8-iso-prostaglandin F2alpha in the first week after Roux-en-Y gastric bypass surgery.* Obesity (Silver Spring), 2011. 19(8): p. 1663-8.

25.     Meng, L.B., et al., *Common Injuries and Repair Mechanisms in the Endothelial Lining.* Chin Med J (Engl), 2018. 131(19): p. 2338-2345.

26.     Satitthummanid, S., et al., *Depleted nitric oxide and prostaglandin E2 levels are correlated with endothelial dysfunction in beta-thalassemia/HbE patients.* Int J Hematol, 2017. 106(3): p. 366-374.

27.	Chistiakov, D.A., A.N. Orekhov, and Y.V. Bobryshev, *Endothelial Barrier and Its Abnormalities in Cardiovascular Disease.* Front Physiol, 2015. 6: p. 365.

28.	Wang, H.H., et al., *Cholesterol and Lipoprotein Metabolism and Atherosclerosis: Recent Advances In reverse Cholesterol Transport.* Ann Hepatol, 2017. 16(0): p. 21-36.

29.	Goldberg, I.J., *Why does diabetes increase atherosclerosis? I don't know!* Journal of Clinical Investigation, 2004. 114(5): p. 613-615.

30.	Hartvigsen, K., et al., *A diet-induced hypercholesterolemic murine model to study atherogenesis without obesity and metabolic syndrome.* Arteriosclerosis Thrombosis and Vascular Biology, 2007. 27(4): p. 878-885.

31.	Wu, L., et al., *Addition of dietary fat to cholesterol in the diets of LDL receptor knockout mice: effects on plasma insulin, lipoproteins, and atherosclerosis.* J Lipid Res, 2006. 47(10): p. 2215-22.

32.	Camare, C., et al., *Angiogenesis in the atherosclerotic plaque.* Redox Biol, 2017. 12: p. 18-34.

33.	Badimon, L. and G. Vilahur, *Thrombosis formation on atherosclerotic lesions and plaque rupture.* J Intern Med, 2014. 276(6): p. 618-32.

34.	Virmani, R., et al., *Lessons from sudden coronary death: a comprehensive morphological classification scheme for atherosclerotic lesions.* Arterioscler Thromb Vasc Biol, 2000. 20(5): p. 1262-75.

35.     Goldberg, I.J., et al., *Decreased lipoprotein clearance is responsible for increased cholesterol in LDL receptor knockout mice with streptozotocin-induced diabetes.* Diabetes, 2008. 57(6): p. 1674-1682.

36.     Horton, J.D., J.C. Cohen, and H.H. Hobbs, *PCSK9: a convertase that coordinates LDL catabolism.* Journal of Lipid Research, 2009. 50: p. S172-S177.

37.     Canuel, M., et al., *Proprotein Convertase Subtilisin/Kexin Type 9 (PCSK9) Can Mediate Degradation of the Low Density Lipoprotein Receptor-Related Protein 1 (LRP-1).* Plos One, 2013. 8(5).

38.     Gimbrone, M.A., Jr. and G. Garcia-Cardena, *Endothelial Cell Dysfunction and the Pathobiology of Atherosclerosis.* Circ Res, 2016. 118(4): p. 620-36.

39.     Tousoulis, D., et al., *The role of nitric oxide on endothelial function.* Curr Vasc Pharmacol, 2012. 10(1): p. 4-18.

40.     Davignon, J. and P. Ganz, *Role of endothelial dysfunction in atherosclerosis.* Circulation, 2004. 109(23 Suppl 1): p. III27-32.

41.     Fan, J.L., et al., *Role of endothelin-1 in atherosclerosis.* Atherosclerosis V: The Fifth Saratoga Conference, 2000. 902: p. 84-94.

42.     Rajwani, A., R.M. Cubbon, and S.B. Wheatcroft, *Cell-specific insulin resistance: implications for atherosclerosis.* Diabetes Metab Res Rev, 2012. 28(8): p. 627-34.

43.     Rask-Madsen, C., et al., *Loss of insulin signaling in vascular endothelial cells accelerates atherosclerosis in apolipoprotein E null mice.* Cell Metab, 2010. 11(5): p. 379-89.

44.    Aveleira, C., *et al, TNF-α Signals Through PKCζ/NF-κB to Alter the Tight Junction Complex and Increase Retinal Endothelial Cell Permeability. Diabetes, 2020.*

45.    Golden SH, Folsom AR, Coresh J, Sharrett AR, Szklo M, Brancati F. Risk factor groupings related to insulin resistance and their synergistic effects on subclinical atherosclerosis: the atherosclerosis risk in communities study. Diabetes. 2002 Oct;51(10):3069-76. doi: 10.2337/diabetes.51.10.3069. PMID: 12351449.

46.    Di Pino A, DeFronzo RA. *Insulin Resistance and Atherosclerosis: Implications for Insulin-Sensitizing Agents.* Endocr Rev. 2019 Dec 1;40(6):1447-1467. doi: 10.1210/er.2018-00141. PMID: 31050706; PMCID: PMC7445419.

47.    Biddinger SB, Hernandez-Ono A, Rask-Madsen C, Haas JT, Alemán JO, Suzuki R, Scapa EF, Agarwal C, Carey MC, Stephanopoulos G, Cohen DE, King GL, Ginsberg HN, Kahn CR. *Hepatic insulin resistance is sufficient to produce dyslipidemia and susceptibility to atherosclerosis.* Cell Metab. 2008 Feb;7(2):125-34. doi: 10.1016/j.cmet.2007.11.013. PMID: 18249172; PMCID: PMC4251554.

48.    Li W, Mclntye TM, Silverstein Rl, *Ferric chloride-induced murine carotid arteria injury: A model of redox pathology.* Redox Biology, Volume 1, Issue 1, 2013

49.    Li W, Nieman M, Gupta AS, *Ferric chloride-induced murine thrombosis models.* J Vis Exp. 2016.

**Tables and Figures**

**Table 1: qRT-PCR analysis of *Ceacam1* mRNA in primary cells**

| | *VECadCre– Cc1$^{+/+}$* | *VECadCre+ Cc1$^{+/+}$* | *VECadCre– Cc1$^{fl/fl}$* | *VECadCre+ Cc1$^{fl/fl}$* |
|---|---|---|---|---|
| Hepatocytes | 4.48 ± 1.13 | 3.99 ± 0.40 | 4.22 ±0.78 | 4.62 ± 1.03 |
| Heart endothelial cells | 2.09 ± 0.12 | 1.96 ± 0.15 | 1.97 ± 0.08 | Negl |
| Hepatic endothelial cells | 2.47 ± 0.15 | 2.52 ± 0.10 | 2.62 ± 0.05 | Negl |
| Macrophages | 1.09 ± 0.09 | 1.31 ± 0.07 | 0.96 ± 0.02 | 1.08 ± 0.15 |
| Hepatic stellate cells | 1.00 ± 0.06 | 0.83 ± 0.05 | 0.79 ± 0.08 | 0.91 ± 0.08 |

Primary cells were isolated from male mice at 2 months of age (n=5/genotype), except for hepatic stellate cells that were derived from male mice at 8 months of age. *Ceacam1* mRNA levels were analyzed by qRT-PCR in triplicate and normalized to 18S. Values are expressed as mean ± SEM. Negl, negligible.

**Table 2: Plasma and tissue biochemistry in 9-month-old male mice propagated on C57BL/6J genetic background**

|  | $VECad-$ $Ccl^{+/+}$ | $VECad+$ $Ccl^{+/+}$ | $VECad-$ $Ccl^{fl/fl}$ | $VECad+$ $Ccl^{fl/fl}$ |
|---|---|---|---|---|
| Body Weight (BW) (g) | $28.4 \pm 0.4$ | $28.3 \pm 0.3$ | $29.2 \pm 0.3$ | $29.3 \pm 0.3$ |
| % WAT/BW | $2.0 \pm 0.2$ | $2.0 \pm 0.2$ | $2.0 \pm 0.2$ | $2.1 \pm 0.2$ |
| Plasma NEFA (mEq/l) | $0.8 \pm 0.1$ | $0.8 \pm 0.1$ | $0.8 \pm 0.2$ | $0.8 \pm 0.2$ |
| Plasma adiponectin (ng/ml) | $33.5 \pm 3.8$ | $30.8 \pm 0.7$ | $28.2 \pm 3.1$ | $30.9 \pm 1.0$ |
| Plasma insulin (pmol/l) | $80.4 \pm 6.1$ | $80.9 \pm 4.5$ | $90.5 \pm 3.4$ | $87.3 \pm 5.9$ |
| Plasma C-peptide ($\times 10^1$ pmol/l) | $20.1 \pm 2.1$ | $20.0 \pm 2.0$ | $20.6 \pm 2.5$ | $20.3 \pm 2.4$ |
| Plasma C/I molar ratio | $4.9 \pm 0.4$ | $5.0 \pm 1.0$ | $5.2 \pm 0.5$ | $5.2 \pm 0.6$ |
| Fasting blood glucose (mg/dl) | $80 \pm 3$ | $82 \pm 3$ | $79 \pm 4$ | $81 \pm 3$ |
| Fed blood glucose (mg/dl) | $101 \pm 2$ | $105 \pm 2$ | $102 \pm 3$ | $104 \pm 3$ |
| Hepatic TG (µg/mg protein) | $54.3 \pm 2.9$ | $59.9 \pm 3.8$ | $60.4 \pm 4.8$ | $54.4 \pm 5.1$ |
| Plasma TG (mg/dl) | $69.0 \pm 3.9$ | $70.2 \pm 4.2$ | $72.8 \pm 4.5$ | $69.8 \pm 4.5$ |
| Plasma HDL-C (mg/dl) | $78.3 \pm 4.0$ | $77.7 \pm 3.0$ | $78.3 \pm 4.2$ | $75.0 \pm 3.9$ |
| Plasma LDL-C (mg/dl) | $24.4 \pm 1.6$ | $23.6 \pm 1.3$ | $24.2 \pm 1.9$ | $24.2 \pm 1.7$ |
| Plasma VLDL-C (mg/dl) | $10.2 \pm 0.6$ | $9.9 \pm 0.6$ | $9.6 \pm 0.3$ | $9.9 \pm 0.5$ |
| Plasma FC (mg/dl) | $52.5 \pm 3.3$ | $53.4 \pm 2.3$ | $50.6 \pm 2.7$ | $53.3 \pm 2.3$ |
| Plasma Total-C (mg/dl) | $99.8 \pm 4.9$ | $98.2 \pm 4.5$ | $98.5 \pm 2.6$ | $102.1 \pm 3.3$ |

Male mice (8-9 months of age, n≥5/genotype) were fasted from 5:00 p.m. until 11:00 a.m. the next morning before blood was drawn and tissues were excised. Fed blood glucose was drawn from randomly fed mice about 3-4 hours of the beginning of the dark cycle. Values are expressed as mean±SEM. % WAT/BW denotes visceral adiposity; steady-state C/I molar ratio is a measure of insulin clearance. -C denotes cholesterol; FC denotes free cholesterol.

**Table 3: Plasma and Tissue Biochemistry in 9-Month-Old Mice Propagated on the C57BL6.*Ldlr*$^{-/-}$ Background and Fed a HC Diet for 3Months**

| | VECad-Ccl$^{+/+}$ | VECad+Ccl$^{+/+}$ | VECad-Ccl$^{fl/fl}$ | VECad+Ccl$^{fl/fl}$ |
|---|---|---|---|---|
| Body weight (g) | 41.5 ± 1.9 | 43.8 ± 1.9 | 40.0 ± 1.4 | 42.1 ± 1.8 |
| % Visceral fat (WAT/BW) | 4.6 ± 0.5 | 4.3 ± 0.5 | 3.9 ± 0.5 | 4.2 ± 0.2 |
| Fasting blood glucose (mg/dl) | 110 ± 9 | 108 ± 7 | 115 ± 15 | 104 ± 8 |
| Fed blood glucose (mg/dl) | 120 ± 7 | 108 ± 9 | 116 ± 5 | 132 ± 5 |
| **Plasma insulin** | | | | |
| Plasma Insulin (pM) | 22.9 ± 3.8 | 19.1 ± 1.0 | 18.9 ± 2.7 | 23.3 ± 1.8 |
| Plasma C-peptide (pM) | 376.8 ± 47.3 | 342.5 ± 28.9 | 343.1 ± 39.5 | 341.1 ± 29.3 |
| Plasma C/I molar ratio | 11.2 ± 3.8 | 12.4 ± 2.5 | 13.8 ± 1.8 | 11.9 ± 2.1 |
| **Hepatic lipid** | | | | |
| Triacylglycerol (μg/mg protein) | 86 ± 11 | 83 ± 5 | 80 ± 6 | 87 ± 3 |
| HMGCR (x10$^3$) | 22 ± 1 | 22 ± 1 | 21 ± 3 | 23 ± 1 |
| **Plasma lipid** | | | | |
| NEFA (mEq/l x10$^{-2}$) | 28 ± 3 | 28 ± 1 | 28 ± 3 | 25 ± 2 |
| Triacylglycerol (mg/dl) | 69 ± 2 | 67 ± 6 | 69 ± 3 | 67 ± 6 |
| Total Cholesterol (mg/dl) | 685 ± 26 | 686 ± 36 | 596 ± 15 | 1043 ± 38*†§ |
| Free Cholesterol (mg/dl) | 151 ± 8 | 155 ± 8 | 149 ± 4 | 152 ± 13 |
| VLDL-C (mg/dl) | 130 ± 1 | 130 ± 3 | 135 ± 1 | 130 ± 1 |
| LDL-C (mg/dl) | 184 ± 3 | 169 ± 9 | 179 ± 9 | 234 ± 3*†§ |
| HDL-C (mg/dl) | 85 ± 3 | 87 ± 3 | 85 ± 3 | 88 ± 4 |
| PCSK9 (pg/ml) | 262 ± 8 | 241 ± 11 | 251 ± 8 | 338 ± 3*†§ |
| ApoB100 (ng/ml) | 368 ± 25 | 455 ± 62 | 395 ± 63 | 1872 ± 137*†§ |
| ApoB48 (μg/ml) | 1907 ± 35 | 1765 ± 50 | 1828 ± 102 | 1790 ± 81 |

Male mice (6 months of age, n>7/genotype) were fed a high-cholesterol diet (HC) for 3 months before sacrifice. Except for fed blood glucose level that was assessed in blood drawn at 10:00 pm, mice were fasted overnight from 5:00 pm until 11:00 am, the next day retro-orbital blood was drawn and tissues were collected. Visceral adiposity: % of gonadal plus inguinal white adipose tissue per body mass; steady-state plasma C-peptide/insulin (C/I) molar ratio was calculated as a measure of insulin clearance; NEFA: non-esterified fatty acids. Plasma VLDL-C was calculated as triacylglycerolx0.2. Data were analyzed by one-way ANOVA with Tukey's for multiple comparisons and values are expressed as mean ± SEM. *P<0.05 *vs* VECad-Ccl$^{+/+}$, †P<0.05 vs VECad+Ccl$^{+/+}$, §P<0.05 vs VECad-Ccl$^{fl/fl}$

**Table S1: Real-time PCR Primer Sequences from Mouse Genes**

| Primer | Forward Sequence (5'-3') | Reverse Sequence (5'-3') |
|---|---|---|
| *Tlr-2* | TTGCTGGGCTGACTTCTCTCA | GAAGAGTCAGGTGATGGATGTCG |
| *Tlr-4* | TCAGAACTTCAGTGGCTGGATT | AACTCTGGATAGGGTTTCCTGTCA |
| *Vcam-1* | ATTTTCTGGGGCAGGAAGTT | ACGTGAGAACAACCGAATCC |
| *Icam-1* | CAATTTCTCATGCCGCACAG | AGCTGGAAGATCGAAAGTCCG |
| *Il-1β* | CCCTGCAGCTGGAGAGTGTGG | TATTCTGTCCATTGAGGTGGAG |
| *Il-6* | CTTGGGACTGCCGCTGGTGA | TGCAAGTGCATCATCGTTGT |
| *Il-4* | AGGTCACAGGAGAAGGGACGCC | TGCGAAGCACCTTGGAAGCCC |
| *Il-13* | TGTTTCGCCACGGCCCCTTC | TGCTCAAGCTGCTGCCTGCC |
| *Il-10* | CACAAAGCAGCCTTGCAGAA | AGAGCAGGCAGCATAGCAGTG |
| *F4/80* | CAAGGAGGACAGAGTTTATCGTG | CTTTGGCTATGGGCTTCCAGTC |
| *Cd4* | TCACCTGGAAGTTCTCTGACC | GGAATCAAAACGATCAAACTGCG |
| *Cd8* | CTCTGGCTGGTCTTCAGTATGA | TCTTTGCCGTATGGTTGGTTT |
| *Cd11β* | TACGTAATTGGGGTGGGAA | GTGCCCTCAATTGCAAAGAT |
| *Mcp-1* | CTTCTGGGCCTGCTGTTCA | CCAGCCTACTCATTGGGATCA |
| *Foxp3* | CCCAGGAAAGACAGCAACCTT | TTTCACAACCAGGCCACTTG |
| *Ctgf* | AATGTCAGTGCGCAGCCGAAGCA | AGGGGTCACGCTCCGTACACAG |
| *Fibronectin* | ACGGTGTCAACTACAAGATCG | GTCTTCCCATCGTCATAGCAC |
| *Col6α3* | GTCAGCTGAGTCTTGTGCTGT | ACCTAGAGAACGTTACCTCACT |
| *α-Sma* | CGTGGCTATTCCTTCGTTAC | TGCCAGGAGACTCCATCC |
| *Tgfβ* | GTGGAAATCAACGGGATCAG | ACTTCCAACCCAGGTCCTTC |
| *Smad7* | GTTGCTGTGAATCTTACGGG | ATCTGGACAGCCTGCA |
| *Et-1* | GGTGGAAGGAAGGAAACTAC | CAAGAAGAGGCAGAAAGGCA |
| *Etar* | AACAAGTGTATGAGGACGGC | GGCCAAGATGAAGGAAAGAA |
| *Etbr* | CAGTCTTCTGCCTGGTCCTC | GGACTGCTTTTCCTCAAACG |
| *eNos* | TCCGGAAGGCGTTTGATC | GCCAAATGTGCTGGTCACC |

| Gp91 | TATGCTGATCCTGCTGCCAGT | TGTCTTCGAATCCTTGTCGAGC |
| Tnfα | CCACCACGCTCTTCTGTCTAC | AGGGTCTGGGCCATAGAACT |
| Nox1 | TTACACGAGAGAAATTCTTGGG | TCGACACACAGGAATCAGGA |
| Nox4 | TCCAAGCTCATTTCCCACAG | CGGAGTTCCATTACATCAGAGG |
| Npc-1 | GGGGCATCAGTTACAATGCT | AAACACCGCACTTCCCATAG |
| Ang-1 | CTCGTCAGACATTCATCATCCA | CACCTTCTTTAGTGCAAAGGCT |
| Ang-2 | CAGCCACGGTCAACAACTC | CTTCTTTACGGATAGCAACCGAG |
| Vegf-A | GCACATAGAGAGAATGAGCTTC | CTCCGCTCTGAACAAGGCT |
| Vegfr-1 | TGGCTCTACGACCTTAGACTG | CAGGTTTGACTTGTCTGAGGTT |
| Vegfr-2 | TTTGGCAAATACAACCCTTCAG | GCAGAAGATACTGTCACCACC |
| VE-Cadherin | CACTGCTTTGGGAGCCTTC | GGGGCAGCGATTCATTTTTCT |
| β-Catenin | TCCCTGAGACGCTAGATGAGG | CGTTTAGCAGTTTTGTCAGCTC |
| Pcsk9 | CAGGGAGCACATTGCATCC | TGCAAAATCAAGGAGCATGGG |
| Lrp1 | GACCAGGTGTTGGACACAGATG | AGTCGTTGTCTCCGTCACACTTC |
| Zo-1 | ACAAACAGCCCTACCAACC | CCATCCTCATCTTCATCTTCTTC |
| Claudin-1 | TGAGCCTCAGAAAAGAGCC | GCCACTAATATCGCCAGACC |
| Claudin-5 | ATGGCGATTACGACAAGAAG | ACTGAGCAAATTCTTGCCC |
| Occludin | CTTCTGCTTCATCGCTTCC | CTTGCCCTTTCCTGCTTTC |
| 18S | TTCGAACGTCTGCCCTATCAA | ATGGTAGGCACGGCGACTA |

**Table S2: mRNA Levels of Inflammation in the Aortae of 9-Month-Old Mice Propagated on the C57BL6.*Ldlr*<sup>-/-</sup> Background and Fed a HC Diet**

| | *VECad-Ccl*$^{+/+}$ | *VECad+Ccl*$^{+/+}$ | *VECad-Ccl*$^{fl/fl}$ | *VECad+Ccl*$^{fl/fl}$ |
|---|---|---|---|---|
| F4/80 | 0.74 ± 0.19 | 0.28 ± 0.07 | 1.20 ± 0.30 | 4.65 ± 1.07*†§ |
| Cd4 | 0.58 ± 0.12 | 0.65 ± 0.11 | 0.64 ± 0.11 | 1.58 ± 0.17*†§ |
| Cd8 | 1.16 ± 0.10 | 1.23 ± 0.13 | 1.07 ± 0.04 | 2.54 ± 0.15*†§ |
| FoxP3 | 0.89 ± 0.05 | 0.82 ± 0.09 | 0.87 ± 0.04 | 0.89 ± 0.06 |
| Il-4 | 0.62 ± 0.15 | 0.96 ± 0.12 | 0.63 ± 0.15 | 0.81 ± 0.06 |
| Il-13 | 0.90 ± 0.45 | 0.92 ± 0.16 | 0.56 ± 0.13 | 0.77 ± 0.17 |
| Il-1β | 0.75 ± 0.06 | 0.72 ± 0.08 | 0.75 ± 0.07 | 1.87 ± 0.23*†§ |
| Il-6 | 0.33 ± 0.09 | 0.53 ± 0.09 | 0.54 ± 0.28 | 1.35 ± 0.25*†§ |
| Tnf-α | 0.35 ± 0.22 | 1.37 ± 0.18 | 1.32 ± 0.90 | 5.50 ± 0.87*†§ |
| Tlr-2 | 0.29 ± 0.18 | 0.39 ± 0.08 | 0.21 ± 0.07 | 2.19 ± 0.69*†§ |
| Tlr-4 | 0.47 ± 0.01 | 0.69 ± 0.12 | 0.52 ± 0.08 | 1.71 ± 0.18*†§ |
| Mcp-1 | 1.19 ± 0.04 | 1.18 ± 0.13 | 1.58 ± 0.16 | 2.59 ± 0.19*†§ |
| Cd11b | 0.93 ± 0.05 | 1.03 ± 0.24 | 1.04 ± 0.07 | 2.31 ± 0.14*†§ |
| Vcam-1 | 0.72 ± 0.27 | 0.75 ± 0.08 | 0.38 ± 0.08 | 2.94 ± 0.65*†§ |

6 months old ldlr$^{-/-}$VECad+Ccl$^{fl/fl}$ mice and their controls (n>5 per group) after 3 months of high cholesterol diet were fasted overnight and sacrificed the next day. Aortae were collected to measure mRNA content by qRT-PCR (normalized to 18s). Values are expressed as mean ± SEM. *P<0.05 *vs* VECad-Ccl$^{+/+,}$ †P<0.05 vs VECad+Ccl$^{+/+}$, §P<0.05 vs VECad-Ccl$^{fl/fl}$

**Table S3: mRNA Levels of Genes in the Aortae of 9-Month-Old Mice Propagated on the C57BL6.*Ldlr*$^{-/-}$ Background and Fed a HC Diet for 3Months**

| | *VECad-Ccl*$^{+/+}$ | *VECad+Ccl*$^{+/+}$ | *VECad-Ccl*$^{fl/fl}$ | *VECad+Ccl*$^{fl/fl}$ |
|---|---|---|---|---|
| ***Tight Junctions*** | | | | |
| Zo-1 | 2.18 ± 0.40 | 2.37 ± 0.18 | 2.11 ± 0.33 | 0.84 ± 0.14*†§ |
| Claudin1 | 2.32 ± 0.11 | 2.07 ± 0.15 | 2.01 ± 0.38 | 0.78 ± 0.04*†§ |
| Claudin5 | 2.06 ± 0.25 | 2.08 ± 0.16 | 2.03 ± 0.37 | 0.69 ± 0.26*†§ |
| Occludin | 2.28 ± 0.05 | 2.89 ± 0.32 | 2.45 ± 0.08 | 0.61 ± 0.06*†§ |
| ***Vascular integrity*** | | | | |
| VE-Cadherin | 1.31 ± 0.12 | 1.23 ± 0.18 | 1.59 ± 0.39 | 0.50 ± 0.05*†§ |
| β-Catenin | 1.05 ± 0.04 | 1.29 ± 0.26 | 1.09 ± 0.12 | 0.48 ± 0.07*†§ |
| Vegf-A | 3.26 ± 0.43 | 3.65 ± 0.41 | 3.29 ± 0.28 | 1.57 ± 0.28*†§ |
| Vegfr-1 | 2.70 ± 0.57 | 2.54 ± 0.42 | 2.31 ± 0.09 | 0.84 ± 0.23*†§ |
| Vegfr-2 | 1.60 ± 0.29 | 1.84 ± 0.14 | 1.29 ± 0.067 | 0.30 ± 0.14*†§ |
| Ang-1 | 2.33 ± 0.49 | 2.11 ± 0.11 | 2.67 ± 0.41 | 0.86 ± 0.04*†§ |
| Ang-2 | 1.36 ± 0.17 | 1.49 ± 0.19 | 1.55 ± 0.31 | 0.27 ± 0.16*†§ |
| ***Oxidative stress*** | | | | |
| Nox4 | 2.40 ± 0.05 | 2.98 ± 0.27 | 2.34 ± 0.42 | 4.52 ± 0.07*†§ |
| Gp91 | 1.32 ± 0.12 | 1.467 ± 0.38 | 2.37 ± 0.51 | 4.16 ± 0.49*†§ |
| Npc-1 | 1.08 ± 0.09 | 1.09 ± 0.11 | 1.05 ± 0.12 | 0.62 ±0.07*†§ |
| ***Fibrosis*** | | | | |
| Fibronectin | 1.44 ± 0.24 | 1.55 ± 0.29 | 0.98 ± 0.16 | 5.14 ± 0.29*†§ |
| Ctgf | 1.41 ± 0.15 | 1.41 ± 0.08 | 1.14 ± 0.26 | 5.53 ± 1.20*†§ |
| Smad7 | 1.49 ± 0.14 | 1.58 ± 0.23 | 1.82 ± 0.39 | 0.54 ± 0.01*†§ |
| Tgf-β | 0.80 ± 0.08 | 0.48 ± 0.41 | 0.94 ± 0.10 | 5.04 ± 0.29*†§ |
| α-Sma | 1.94 ± 0.32 | 2.13 ± 0.30 | 1.34 ± 0.33 | 7.25 ± 1.21*†§ |
| Col6- α3 | 1.29 ± 0.11 | 1.29 ± 0.13 | 1.53 ± 0.27 | 3.14 ± 0.06*†§ |
| Et-1 | 1.75 ± 0.65 | 1.04 ± 0.20 | 1.30 ± 0.13 | 3.30 ± 0.29*†§ |
| Etar | 1.05 ± 0.20 | 0.89 ± 0.40 | 1.04 ± 0.49 | 3.44 ± 0.41*†§ |
| Etbr | 2.36 ± 0.51 | 2.19 ± 0.17 | 2.14 ± 0.23 | 0.76 ± 0.10*†§ |
| Etar/ Etbr | 0.64 ± 0.20 | 0.22 ± 0.07 | 0.60 ± 0.27 | 3.10 ± 0.85*†§ |

6 months old ldlr$^{-/-}$VECad+Ccl$^{fl/fl}$ male mice and their controls (n>5 per group) after 3 months of high cholesterol diet were fasted overnight and sacrificed the next day. Aortae were collected to measure mRNA content by qRT-PCR (normalized to 18s). Values are expressed as mean ± SEM. *P<0.05 *vs* VECad-Ccl$^{+/+}$, †P<0.05 vs VECad+Ccl$^{+/+}$, §P<0.05 vs VECad-Ccl$^{fl/fl}$

## A. Body weight and daily food intake of C57BL6 mice

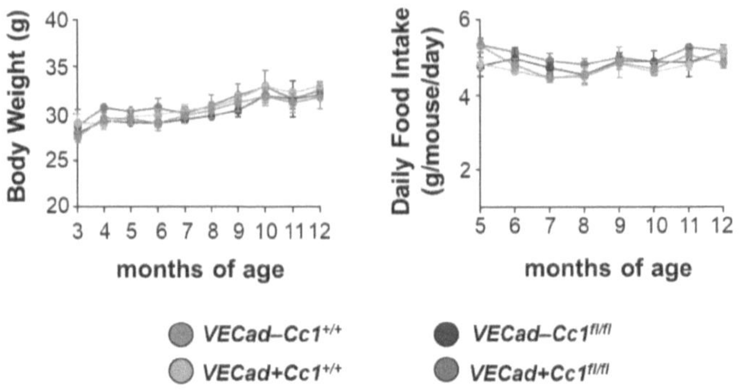



## B. Intraperitoneal insulin/glucose tolerance in C57BL6 mice

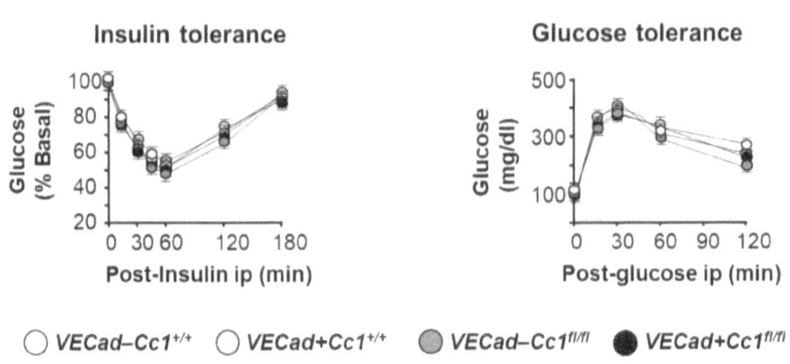

## A. En-face of aortae in C57BL6 mice

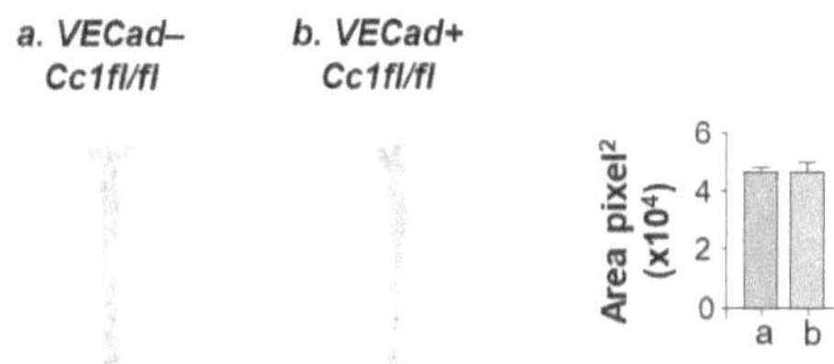


## B. Aortic root staining in C57BL6 mice

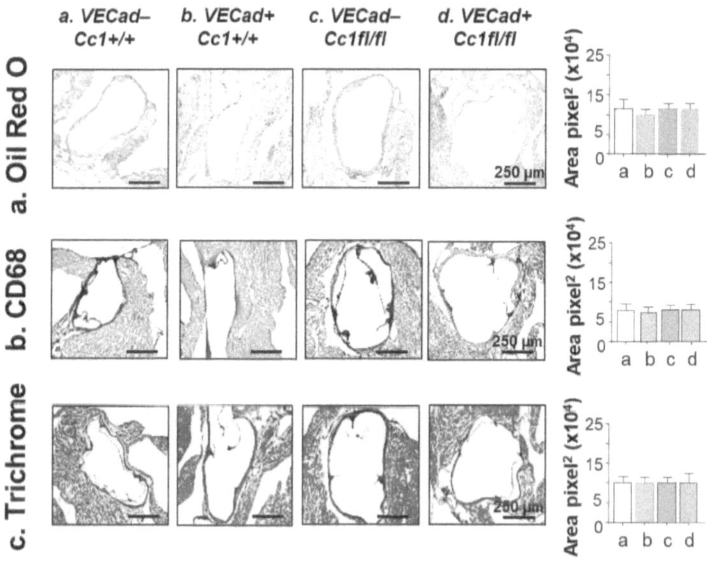

## A. Body Weight

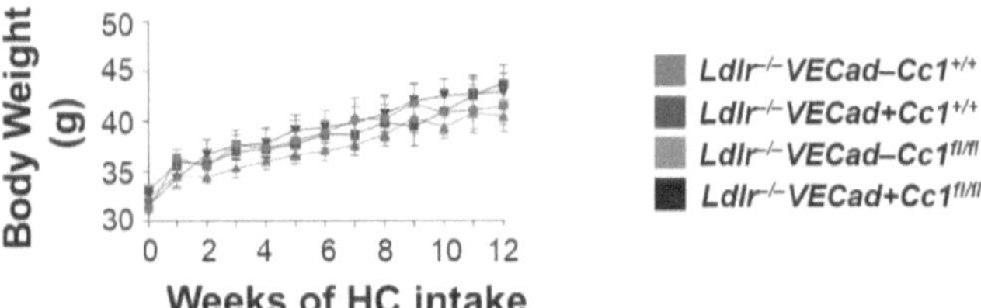


## B. Insulin tolerance

## C. Glucose tolerance

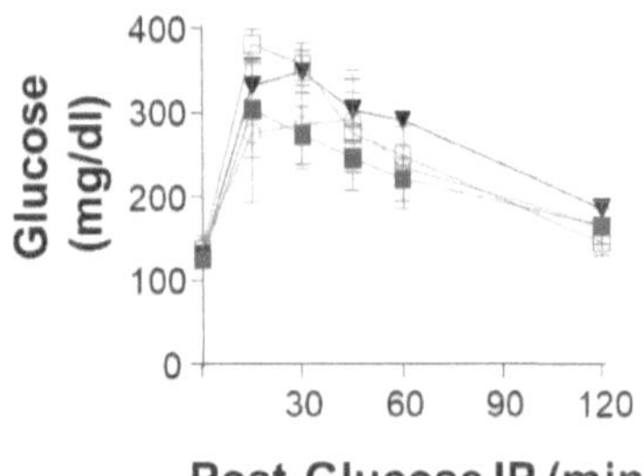

## A. En-face of aortic lesions in *Ldlr*−/− mice on HC for 5 months

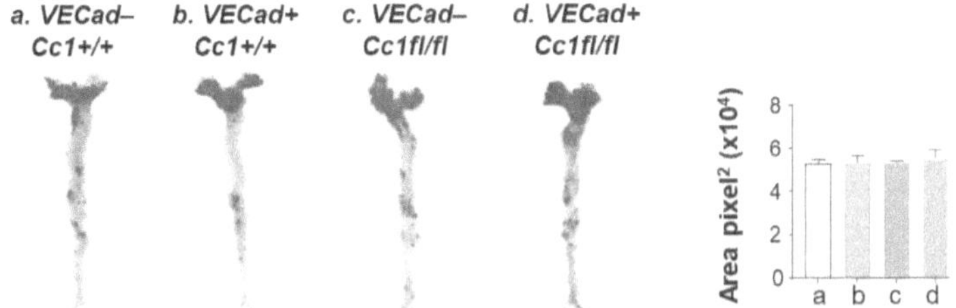


## B. Plasma cholesterol levels in *Ldlr*−/− mice on HC for 5 months

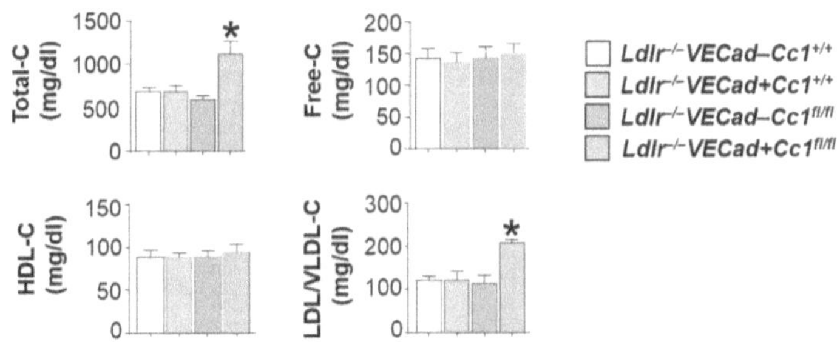


## C. Oil red-O staining of aortic roots in *Ldlr*−/− mice fed HC for 3 months

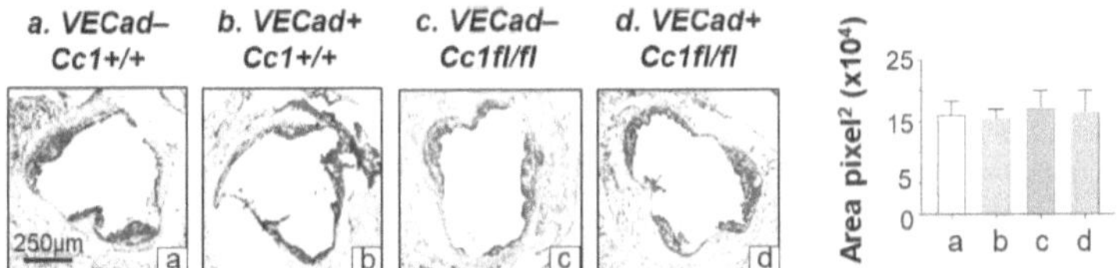

## A. IHC of CD68 in aortic root in *Ldlr*<sup>-/-</sup> mice on HC for 5 months

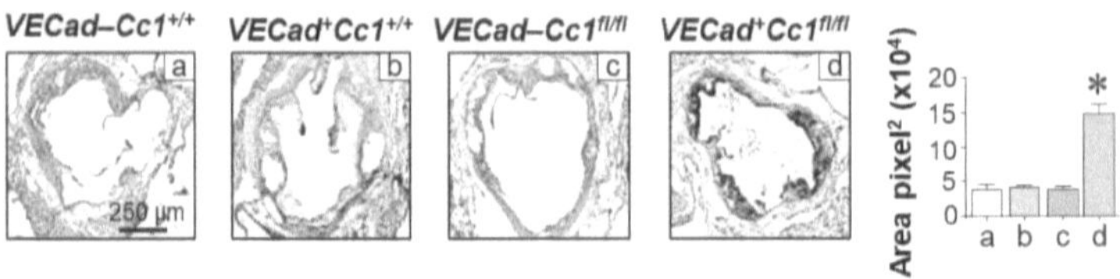


## B. Plasma levels of cytokines in *Ldlr*<sup>-/-</sup> mice

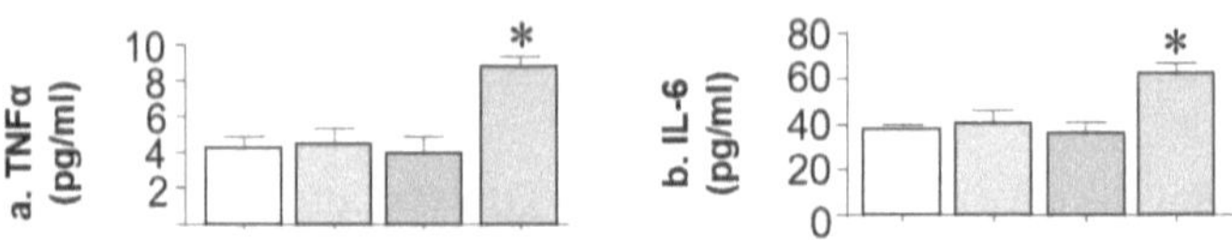


## C. Western analysis in aorta in *Ldlr*<sup>-/-</sup> mice

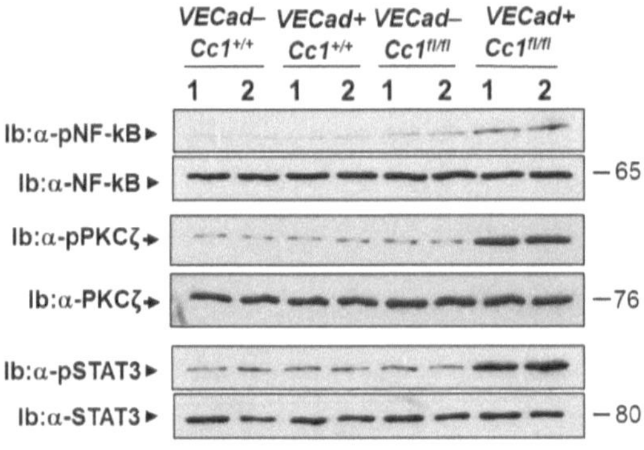

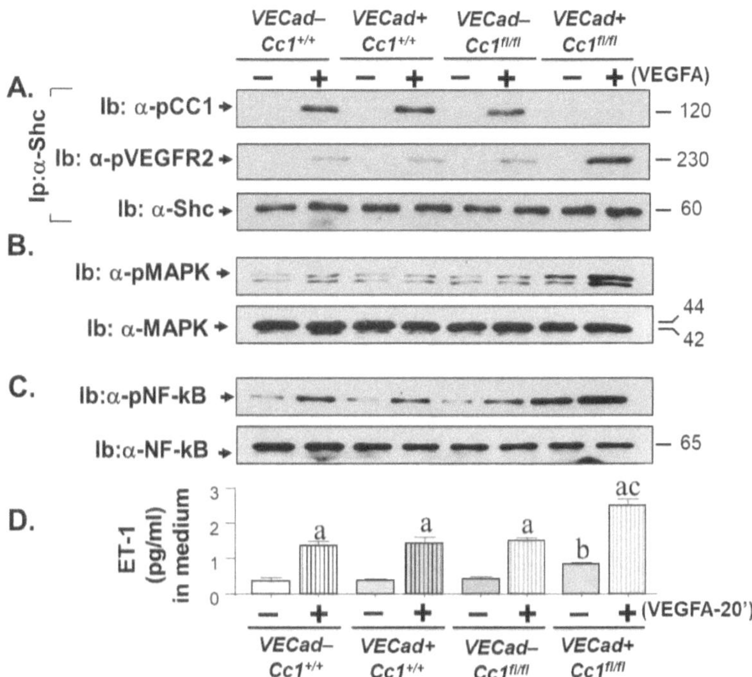


## E. Plasma pro-fibrogenic factors in *Ldlr*−/− mice fed HC for 3 months

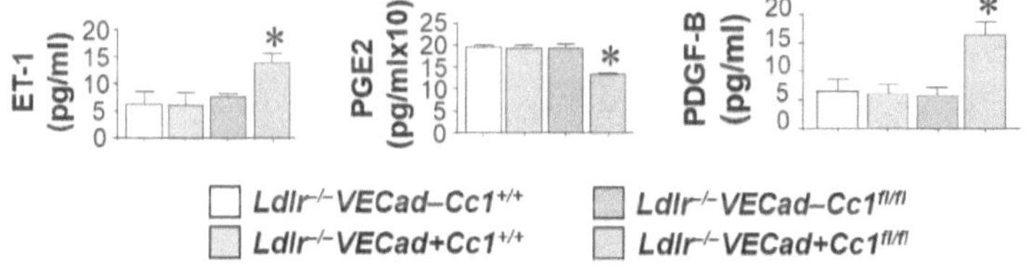

## A. Evans blue: Vascular permeability in *Ldlr*⁻/⁻ mice

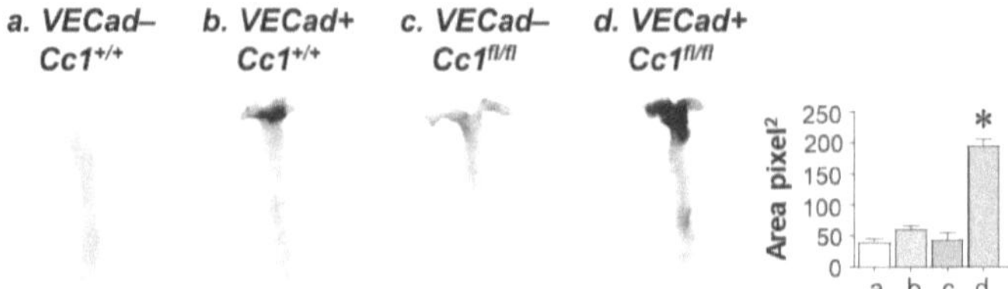


## B. Western blot analysis of *Ldlr*⁻/⁻ aortae

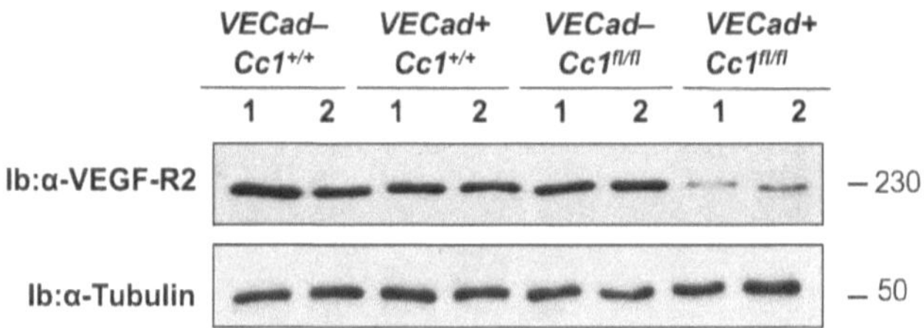


## C. Intravital microscopy of leukocyte adhesion in carotid artery of *Ldlr*⁻/⁻ mice

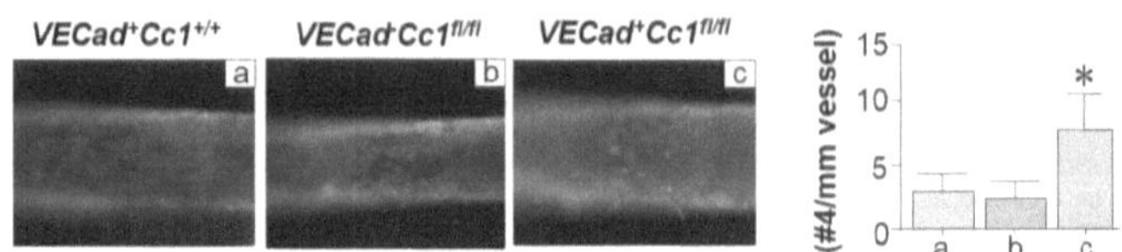

## A. Plasma levels of redox parameters in *Ldlr⁻ᐟ⁻* mice fed HC for 3 months

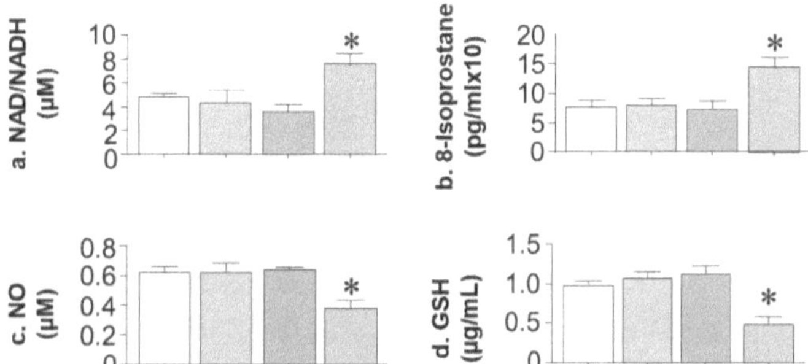


## B. NO level in aortae of *Ldlr⁻ᐟ⁻* mice

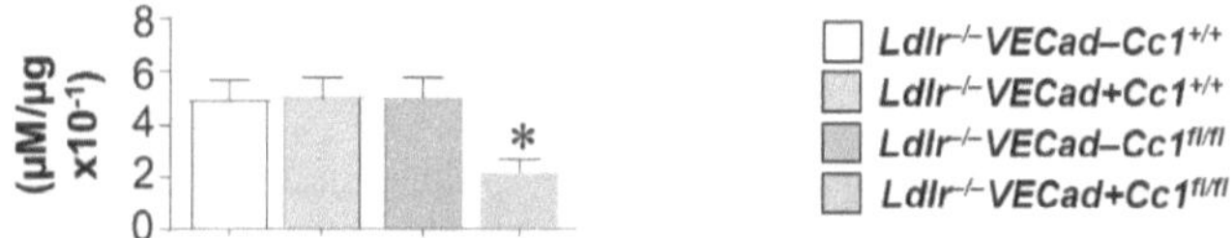

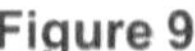


Figure 9 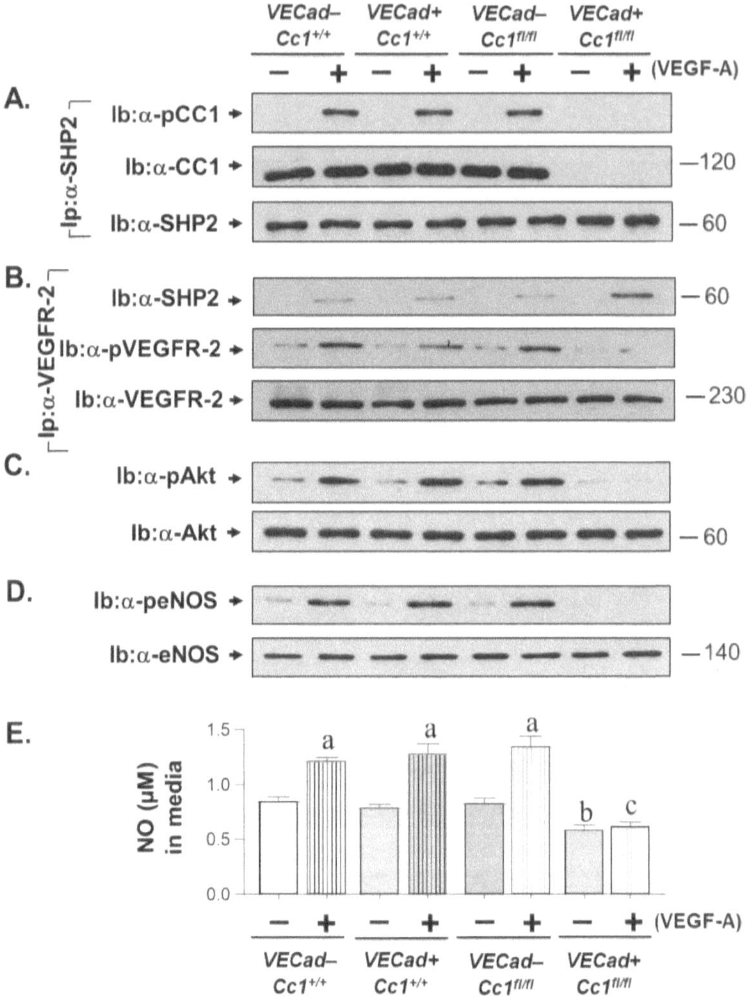
VECad– VECad+ VECad– VECad+
Cc1+/+ Cc1+/+ Cc1fl/fl Cc1fl/fl
− + − + − + − + (VEGF-A)
A.
Ip:α-SHP2
Ib:α-pCC1
Ib:α-CC1 —120
Ib:α-SHP2 —60
B.
Ip:α-VEGFR-2
Ib:α-SHP2 —60
Ib:α-pVEGFR-2
Ib:α-VEGFR-2 —230
C.
Ib:α-pAkt
Ib:α-Akt —60
D.
Ib:α-peNOS
Ib:α-eNOS —140
E.
NO (µM) in media
1.5
1.0
0.5
0.0
a a a
b c
− + − + − + − + (VEGF-A)
VECad– VECad+ VECad– VECad+
Cc1+/+ Cc1+/+ Cc1fl/fl Cc1fl/fl

## A. Trichome staining of aortic roots of *Ldlr*−/− mice on HC in the last 4 months

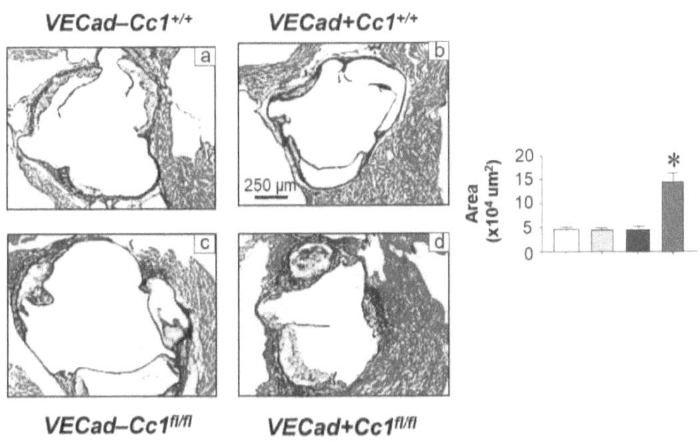



## B. TGFβ signaling in aortae of *Ldlr*−/− mice

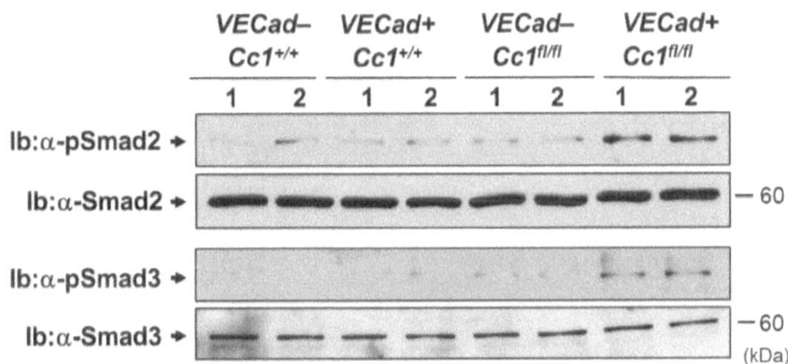

## A. Genotyping of mice using ear lysates

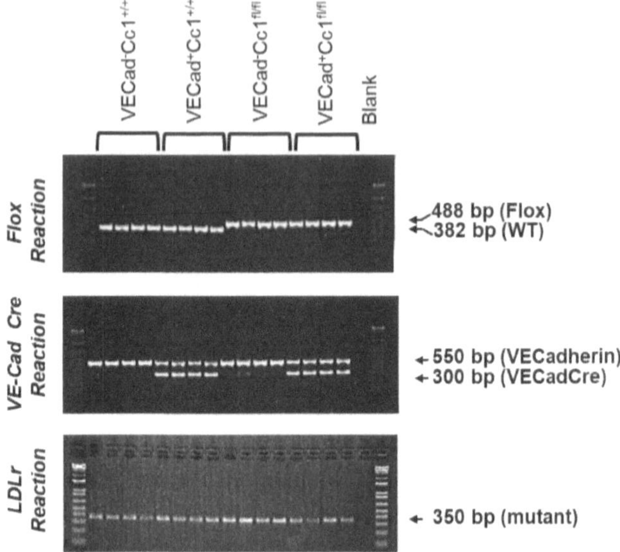



### Primer sequences used for genotyping by Polymerase Chain Reaction

| Gene | ID | Primer sequence (5'-3') |
| --- | --- | --- |
| Flox | Flox A FP | ACACAAGGAGGCCTCTCAGATGGCG |
| | Flox B RP | GACTTTGGCTTCCTGACTGGAGGA |
| | Flox C RP | GCGCCTCCCCTACCCGGTAGAATT |
| Cre | VE-Cadherin Cre FP | GCAGGCAGCTCACAAAGGAACAAT |
| | VE-Cadherin Cre RP | ATCACTCGTTGCATCGACCGGTAA |
| | VE-Cadherin Gene RP | TGTCCTTGCTGAGTGACAGTGGAA |
| Ldlr | OMIR33 49 FP | CCATATGCATCCCCAGTCTT |
| | OMIR33 50 RP | GCGATGGATACACTCACTGC |
| | OMIR00 92 RP | AATCCATCTTGTTCAATGGCCGATC |

## Intraperitoneal Insulin tolerance test in 11- month-old *Ldlr*‑/‑ mice fed a HC diet in the last 5 months

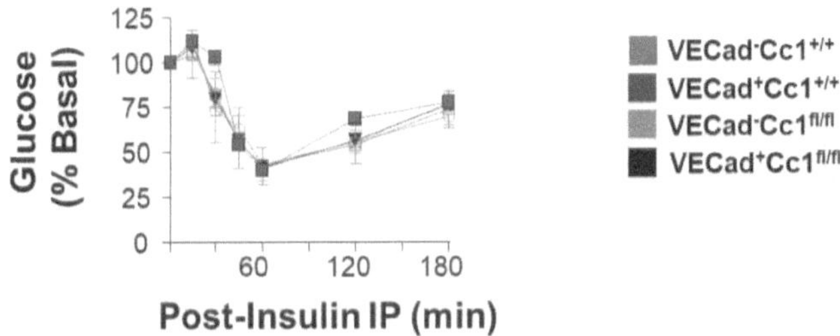

# Chapter 3: Regulation of Hepatic Fibrosis by Carcinoembryonic Antigen-related Cell Adhesion Molecule 1

**Introduction**

Non-alcoholic fatty liver disease (NAFLD) is a complex disease encompassing a cadre of metabolic dysregulation and histological anomalies that include hepatic steatosis without or with inflammation, chicken-wire bridging fibrosis and apoptosis. Combined, these metabolic and molecular events develop into non-alcoholic steatohepatitis (NASH) [113]. The disease is commonly associated with metabolic syndrome in light of their parallel epidemic spread worldwide [114] and of their shared intertwined molecular and cellular mechanisms underlying their pathogenesis. These include, insulin resistance, lipotoxicity, inflammation and oxidative stress [115-118].

Whereas the role of chronic hyperinsulinemia and insulin resistance in NASH pathogenesis remains controversial, it appears to play a critical role in the initiation and early switch from simple steatosis to NAFLD [119, 120]. This provided the impetus to use insulin sensitizers as therapeutic modalities to curb NAFLD in patients with insulin resistance in the absence of an FDA-approved drug specifically targeting advanced fibrosis [121, 122].

Chronic hyperinsulinemia in patients with NAFLD has been attributed to impaired insulin clearance rather than increased insulin secretion [123]. Moreover, insulin-resistant obese subjects with NAFLD manifested reduced hepatic levels of Carcinoembryonic Antigen-Related Cell Adhesion molecule 1 (CEACAM1) [124, 125], a glycoprotein that promotes receptor-mediated insulin uptake and targeting to the degradation process in hepatocytes [64]. Consistently, $Cc1^{-/-}$ mice with global null deletion [126, 127], AlbCre+$Cc1^{fl/fl}$ mice with liver-specific deletion [72] of *Ceacam1* gene, and L-SACC1 mice with liver-specific inactivation of CEACAM1 [128] manifested chronic hyperinsulinemia driven by impaired insulin clearance. This in turn, caused insulin resistance (due to downregulation of the insulin receptor) and hepatic steatosis (owing to increased hyperinsulinemia-driven SREBP-1c activation of lipogenic genes transcription and to the loss of the repression on FASN activity mediated by CEACAM1 [129]). With fatty acid $\Box$-oxidation being compromised, the increase in *de novo* lipogenesis tips the balance towards fat accumulation (hepatic steatosis) and drives its redistribution to white adipose tissue (WAT) for storage (visceral obesity). In agreement with increased inflammatory response to fat accumulation, mice with global deletion of *Ceacam1* ($Ccl^{-/-}$) developed steatohepatitis [130] in the absence of deranged cholesterol homeostasis [131]. Fed a high-fat diet, they also developed a progressive NASH-like phenotype including macro-steatosis and lipid peroxidation in addition to apoptosis and advanced fibrosis [132]. Similarly, liver-specific AlbCre+$Ccl^{fl/fl}$ nulls manifested NASH with advanced fibrosis when propagated on the $Ldlr^{-/-}$ background and fed a cholesterol-enriched diet [133].

Because CEACAM1 is expressed in all liver cells that are virtually implicated in stellate cell activation [134], and in light of the positive role of free cholesterol lipotoxicity in hepatocellular injury [116], the aforementioned loss-of-function models do not efficiently delineate the role of hyperinsulinemia caused by primary deletion of *Ceacam1* in hepatocytes independently of altered cholesterol homeostasis. Because liver-specific reconstitution of CEACAM1 restored insulin clearance and insulin sensitivity in addition to curbing hepatic steatosis in $Ccl^{-/-}$ mice fed a regular chow diet

[90], the current studies investigated whether it can also reverse the advanced fibrogenic NASH phenotype driven by prolonged high-fat feeding in parallel to restoring normoinsulinemia and insulin sensitivity.

**Methods**

*Mice maintenance*

As previously described [90], mice with global deletion of *Ceacam1* gene (C57BL/6J.*Cc1*$^{-/-}$ or *Cc1*$^{-/-}$) were bred with mice harboring liver-specific overexpression of rat *Ceacam1* transgene driven by apolipoprotein-A1 promoter (L-CC1) [135]. Genotyping was performed [25] by PCR analysis (Fig. S1) using rat and mouse specific primers (Fig. S1B). In addition to L-CC1, control littermates include *Cc1*$^{+/+}$ without the transgene. Only male mice were examined. All mice were kept in a 12-hour dark/light cycle and fed *ad libitum* a standard chow (RD) or a 45% high-fat diet (Research Diets, Catalog D12451, New Brunswick, NJ) for three or five months prior to phenotypic analysis. All procedures were approved by the Institutional Animal Care and Utilization Committees at Ohio University and the University of Toledo.

*Insulin and glucose tolerance tests*

Following a 7-hour-fast, mice were injected intraperitoneally with insulin (0.75 U/kg BW, Novo Nordisk) (for insulin tolerance) or glucose (1.5 g/kg BW of 50% dextrose solution, Dextrose Injection, USP) (for glucose tolerance). Blood was drawn from the tail vein at 0-180 min post-injection to measure glucose levels.

*Whole body composition*

This was assessed in live mice by nuclear magnetic resonance (Bruker Minispec, Billerica, MA, USA).

*Metabolic parameters*

Mice were fasted overnight and retro-orbital blood was drawn beginning at 11:00 a.m. the following morning to assess steady-state levels of plasma insulin (Mouse Ultrasensitive ELISA kit, Alpco, Salem, NH), C-peptide (ELISA, Alpco), non-esterified fatty acids (NEFA C kit, Wako Diagnostics, Richmond, VA), triacylglycerol (Pointe Scientific Triglyceride), endothelin-1 (ELISA kit, ab133030, Abcam, Cambridge, MA), TNFα (SimpleStep ELISA kit, ab208348, Abcam) and Il-6 (ELISA Kit, ab222503, Abcam). Hepatic triacylglycerol was measured as previously described [135], hepatic nitric oxide (NO) levels using Nitrate/Nitrite Fluorometric Assay (780051, Cayman Chemical, Ann Arbor, MI), and hepatic levels of reduced glutathione (GSH) were measured using the Bioxytech GSH-400 kit (OXISResearch, Portland, OR). Plasma Alanine Transaminase (ALT) (ab105134, Abcam) and Aspartate Aminotransferase (AST) (ab105135) colorimetric assays kits were used to assess liver function.

*Liver histology*

Hematoxylin-eosin (H&E) was performed on formalin-fixed, paraffin-embedded liver sections. Deparaffinized and rehydrated slides were stained with 0.1% Sirius Red (Sigma, Direct Red 80, St Louis, MO) to assess fibrosis.

*Fatty acid synthase activity*

Frozen livers were homogenized and the supernatant was added to a reaction mix containing 0.1μCi [$^{14}$C] malonyl-coenzyme A (Perkin-Elmer, Akron, OH), as previously described [129]. 1:1 chloroform: methanol solution was added to stop the reaction, and fatty acid synthase activity was calculated as counts/min of [$^{14}$C] incorporated/μg cell lysates.

*Ex vivo palmitate oxidation*

Livers were homogenized before being incubated in 0.2mM of [1-$^{14}$C] palmitate (0.5 mCi/ml) (American Radiolabeled Chemicals, St Louis, MO), as described previously [90]. Perchloric acid was added to stop the reaction and recover the radioactive acid soluble metabolites. Trapped $CO_2$ radioactivity and partial oxidation products were measured using liquid scintillation. The oxidation rate was expressed as the sum of complete and partial fatty acid oxidation expressed in nmoles/g/min.

*Western blot analysis*

Livers were lysed and analyzed by SDS-PAGE followed by immunoprobing with polyclonal antibodies against phospho-Smad2 (Ser465/467), phospho-Smad3 (Ser423/425), Smad-7, α-SMA, CHOP, phospho-Stat3 (Y705), phospho-NF-ĶB (S536), phospho-eNOS (Ser 1177), phospho-PKCζ (phosphothreonine-Thr 410/403) (Cell Signaling, Danvers, MA, and custom-made rabbit polyclonal 3759 against mouse CEACAM1, and custom-made rat CEACAM1 (αP3[Y488]) [25]. For normalization, proteins were probed with polyclonal antibodies against Smad 2, Smad3, Stat3, NF-ĶB, eNOS, PKCζ and Tubulin (Cell Signaling) using parallel gels. Blots were incubated with horseradish peroxidase-conjugated donkey anti-rabbit IgG or sheep anti-mouse IgG antibody (GE Healthcare Life Sciences, Amersham, Marlborough, MA) and proteins were visualized using ECL (Amersham).

*Real-time quantitative RT-PCR*

Total RNA was isolated from livers with NucleoSpin RNA Kit (740955.50, Macherey-Nagel, Bethlehem, PA) and from white adipose tissue using TRIzol Reagent (15596026, Ambion, Life Technologies, CA). cDNA was synthesized by iScript cDNA Synthesis Kit (Bio-Rad Life Science, Hercules, CA), using 1μg of total RNA and oligodT primers. cDNA was evaluated with semi-quantitative RT-PCR (qRT-PCR; StepOne Plus, Applied Biosystems), and mRNA was normalized to GAPDH (for regular diet fed mice), 18S (for high-fat fed mice) or 36B4 (for white adipose tissue regardless of diet). using primers listed in Table S2.

*Statistical analysis*

Data were analyzed by one-way analysis of variance (ANOVA) with Tukey's for multiple comparisons using GraphPad Prism 7 software. $P<0.05$ was considered statistically significant.

**Results**

*Rescuing hepatic CEACAM1 expression in Cc1$^{-/-}$ mice restored insulin clearance and sensitivity in mice fed a high-fat diet*

Western blot analysis detected transgenic rat, but not endogenous mouse CEACAM1 in the livers of $Cc1^{-/-\text{xliver+}}$ rescue mice fed regular chow (RD) or high-fat (HF) diet (Fig. 1A). Using rat- and mouse-specific primers (Fig. S1B and Table S2), qRT-PCR analysis detected mRNA of transgenic rat Ceacam1 in the liver, but not in the hypothalamus, skeletal muscle or white adipose tissue (WAT) of $Cc1^{-/-\text{xliver+}}$ mice (Table S1).

As Table 1 shows, liver-specific reconstitution of *Ceacam1* reversed total fat and plasma NEFA, and restored lean mass in 6-month-old RD-fed $Cc1^{-/-}$ mice (Table 1), as expected from the previously reported effect on 8-month-old mice [25]. It exerted a similar protective effect when mice were fed a high-fat diet for 3 (Table 1) and 5 months (not shown). Consistent with a key role for CEACAM1 in promoting insulin clearance, steady-state C-peptide/insulin molar ratio was lower in RD-fed and HF-diet fed $Cc1^{-/-}$ mice, leading to chronic hyperinsulinemia (Table 1). This leads to insulin resistance [assessed by insulin intolerance (Fig. 1B.*i*) and fed hyperglycemia in RD-fed nulls relative to wild-type controls (Table 1)]. The mutation also caused glucose intolerance (Fig. 1B.*ii*). Insulin resistance provoked a compensatory increase in insulin secretion in RD-fed nulls, as suggested by the higher plasma C-peptide levels relative to controls (Table 1). In contrast to wild-type $Cc1^{+/+}$ and L-CC1 controls, HF caused fasting hyperglycemia in $Cc1^{-/-}$ nulls. Liver-specific redelivery of *Ceacam1* restored insulin clearance to reverse hyperinsulinemia and fed hyperglycemia (Table 1), and normalized insulin and glucose tolerance in RD-fed and HF-fed $Cc1^{-/-\times liver+}$ mice (Fig. 1B). It also reversed diet-induced fasting hyperglycemia (Table 1) even after 5 months of HF intake (119±9 in $Cc1^{-/-\times liver+}$ vs 154±7 in $Cc1^{-/-}$ mice).

*Liver-specific reconstitution of CEACAM1 in null mice reversed diet-induced hepatic steatosis*

Histological analysis of H&E-stained liver sections revealed diffuse microvesicular lipid droplets in the liver parenchyma of RD-fed $Cc1^{-/-}$ mice (Fig. 2A.*iii*) and a mixture of micro- and macrovesicular lipid deposits when fed a HF diet (Fig.

2A.*vii*). This was supported by increased hepatic triglyceride without changes in total cholesterol levels (Table 1). Hepatic restoration of CEACAM1 curbed lipid accumulation in both RD- and HF-fed $Ccl^{-/-xliver+}$ mice (Fig. 2A, *iv* vs *iii* and *viii* vs *vii*). This was supported by its ~1.5-to-2-fold lowering effect on hepatic triglyceride levels (Table 1). Increased hepatic lipid accumulation in RD-fed and HF-fed $Ccl^{-/-}$ mice relative to $Ccl^{+/+}$ and L-CC1 controls stemmed from the combined effect of enhanced fatty acid transport (high CD36 mRNA) in RD-fed (Table S3) and HF-fed null livers (Table S4); increased *de novo* lipogenesis [as demonstrated by higher fatty acid synthase (FASN) activity (Figs. 2B.*i*)] and reduced fatty acid β-oxidation (Figs. 2B.*ii*). Elevated FASN activity in $Ccl^{-/-}$ livers could partly stem from increased hyperinsulinemia-driven transcriptional upregulation by SREBP-1c (Table S3-S4). Reduced hepatic fatty acid β-oxidation (Figs. 2B.*ii*) is consistent with the ~2-fold lower Fgf21 mRNA levels in RD-fed and HF-fed $Ccl^{-/-}$ mice relative to controls (Table S3-S4). Liver-specific reconstitution of CEACAM1 attenuated lipogenesis as indicated by limiting CD36 mRNA levels (Table S3-S4) and normalization of FASN activity (Fig. 2B.*i*) and mRNA levels (Table S3-S4) in response to both diets. It also induced hepatic fatty acid β-oxidation under both feeding conditions (Fig. 2B.*ii*), in part related to recovering Fgf21 expression levels (Table S3-S4, $Ccl^{-/-xliver+}$ vs $Ccl^{-/-}$). This demonstrated that reconstituting hepatic CEACAM1 blunted steatosis by limiting NEFA transport likely via reducing visceral obesity and lipolysis, reducing *de novo* lipogenesis and increasing fatty acid β-oxidation in the livers of $Ccl^{-/-xliver+}$ mice.

*Liver-specific rescuing of CEACAM1 expression in null mice reversed diet-induced hepatic inflammation*

H&E staining revealed a few inflammatory infiltrates in RD-fed $Ccl^{-/-}$ livers with no significant change in hepatocellular architecture (Fig. 2A.*iii*). Consistent with lipotoxicity-driven inflammation, HF feeding increased perivascular and lobular inflammatory cell infiltrates in $Ccl^{-/-}$ livers by comparison to $Ccl^{+/+}$ and L-CC1 controls (Fig. 2A.*vii*). Liver-specific rescuing of CEACAM1 markedly curbed this inflammatory response to HF diet (Fig. 2A.*viii* vs *vii*, Table 3).

qRT-PCR analysis showed an increase in total (F4/80) and activated (Cd68) macrophage pool, and in neutrophil levels (Mpo, Elastase) in null livers relative to $Ccl^{+/+}$ and L-CC1 controls under both feeding conditions (Table S3-S4). Null livers also manifested higher mRNA of pro-inflammatory CD+4 and CD+8 T-lymphocytes with no increase in anti-inflammatory Treg pools (Foxp3 and IL-10) (Table S3-S4). Higher Ifnγ, but not IL-4 and IL-13 mRNA levels in null livers under both feeding conditions (Table S3-S4), indicates a $CD4^{+}Th1$ response. This pro-inflammatory state was marked by the activation of hepatic NF-κB in null mice under both feeding conditions (assessed by immunoblotting liver lysates with α-phospho-NF-κB normalized to loaded NF-κB, Fig. 2C). NF-κB induced the transcription of its targets, including pro-inflammatory cytokines such as TNFα, IL-1β, and IL-6 (Table S3-S4), followed by their release, as manifested by elevated plasma TNFα and IL-6 levels in null mice under both feeding conditions (Table 2). IL-6 could, in turn, activate Stat3-mediated pro-inflammatory pathways (Fig. 2C) to synergize with TNFα activation of NF-κB to induce mRNA levels of Mcp-1/Ccl2 in monocytes/macrophages (Table S3-S4) and amplify their migration. Stat3 activation also represses interferon regulatory factor-8 (Irf-8) expression to upregulate the expression of Cd11b+ macrophages and granulocytes (Gr1 mRNA) (Table S3-S4) [27-29], thereby sustaining a pro-inflammatory state under both feeding conditions. Interestingly, liver-specific reconstitution of CEACAM1 reversed NF-$\kappa$B and Stat3 activation (Fig. 2C), the rise in plasma TNF$\alpha$ and IL-6 and in the mRNA levels of pro-inflammatory cytokines and chemokines (Table S3-S4) under both feeding conditions. This lends further support to the critical role of hepatic CEACAM1 in regulating the inflammatory milieu of the liver [20].

In addition to the liver, HF amplified the activation of macrophages (F4/80, Cd68) and the production of pro-inflammatory cytokines (Tnf$\alpha$, Il-1$\beta$; Il-6) in WAT of null mice (Table S5). This could promote a pro-inflammatory state (elevated plasma TNF$\alpha$ and IL-6) which synergizes with increased NEFA release to cause systemic insulin resistance in $Ccl^{-/-}$ mice compared to WT and L-CC1 controls [30]. Liver-specific reconstitution of CEACAM1 reversed this inflammatory response in WAT under both feeding conditions (Table S5, $Ccl^{-/-xliver+}$ vs $Ccl^{-/-}$).

*Liver-specific redelivery of CEACAM1 in null mice reversed apoptosis, hepatic injury, and oxidative stress caused by high-fat diet*

Both RD-fed and HF-fed $Ccl^{-/-}$ mice manifested liver dysfunction as assessed by their ~2-fold higher plasma alanine transaminase (ALT) and aspartate aminotransferase (AST) levels relative to $Ccl^{+/+}$ and L-CC1 controls (Table 2). Liver-specific reconstitution of CEACAM1 normalized plasma ALT and AST levels and restored liver function in null mice (Table 2).

Apoptosis contributes to cell injury and liver dysfunction. Consistently, Tunel staining detected more apoptotic cells in HF-fed null, but not control livers (Fig. 2D.*iii*). Moreover, mRNA level of *Chop*, an apoptosis marker, was induced by ~3-fold in HF-fed, but not in RD-fed *Ccl*$^{-/-}$ livers (Table S4-S3). This translated into higher hepatic CHOP protein content in HF-fed, but not RD-fed *Ccl*$^{-/-}$ mice (Fig. 2D.*ii*). Together with the ~4-fold decrease in the mRNA levels of the anti-apoptosis Bcl2 gene in HF-fed null mice (Table S4), this pointed to the apoptosis-inducing effect of HF feeding in null livers. qRT-PCR analysis revealed an ~2-to-3-fold increase in the mRNA levels of hepatic injury markers (Hgf, Nqo1, Nrf1) in RD-fed and HF-fed *Ccl*$^{-/-}$ livers (Table S3-S4).

Consistent with oxidative stress contributing to hepatocyte dysfunction [6], hepatic mRNA levels of NADPH oxidase (Nox1 and Nox4) were elevated (Table S3-S4) and hepatic nitric oxide (NO) levels were lower in RD-fed and HF-fed nulls as compared to controls (Table 2), likely due to compromised activation of the Akt/eNOS pathway in null livers, as previously shown [36] and as manifested by reduced basal eNOS phosphorylation (Fig. 2C). Additionally, RD-fed *Ccl*$^{-/-}$ livers manifested normal mRNA levels of Cyp2E1, a cytochrome p450 enzyme involved in the metabolism of long-chain fatty acids (lipooxygenation) and microsomal lipid β-peroxidation (Table S3). HF diet induced Cyp2E1 mRNA by ~2-fold in *Ccl*$^{-/-}$, but not control livers (Table S4 vs S3), possibly by activating NF-κB pathways [31]. Moreover, HF lowered Npc1 mRNA in null livers by ~50%, contributing to reduced GSH levels (Table 2) and subsequently, increased response to the cytotoxic effect of elevated TNFα levels in null mice [32], which could in turn, activate IKK-β, a redox-sensitive kinase that upregulates NF-κB–dependent proinflammatory pathways [33]. In addition, HF, but not RD intake, induced PKC-ζ activation (phosphorylation) in null but not WT mice (Fig. 2C). In light of PKC-ζ activation of NF-κB [34], its preferential phosphorylation in HF-fed null mice could contribute to diet-induced nitroso-redox imbalance and hepatocyte injury in null livers.

Liver-specific reconstitution of CEACAM1 restored liver function even in response to HF intake (assessed by normalizing ALT and AST levels, Table 2). It also reversed HF-induced apoptosis in $Cc1^{-/-xliver+}$ mice [reducing tunel stained cells, restoring Bcl2 and Chop mRNA levels (Table S3) and normalizing CHOP protein content (Fig. 2D)]. It also prevented oxidative stress and liver injury in RD-fed as well as HF-fed nulls ($Cc1^{-/-xliver+}$ vs $Cc1^{-/-}$ mice). This assigns a major role for hepatic CEACAM1-dependent pathways in protecting against hepatocyte injury and apoptosis caused by HF intake.

*Liver-specific reconstitution of CEACAM1 protected against fibrosis in null mice*

Advanced features of NASH include fibrosis in addition to apoptosis. As previously reported [22], Sirius red staining showed spontaneous  and diet-amplified interstitial chicken-wire pattern of collagen deposition in $Cc1^{-/-}$ mice (Fig. 3A). These pathologies were reversed to basal levels of $Cc1^{+/+}$ and L-CC1 controls upon exclusive hepatic rescuing of CEACAM1 (Fig. 3A.*iv* vs *iii and viii vs vii)*. Consistently, mRNA levels of pro-fibrogenic genes (Tgfβ, α-Sma, Ctgf) (Fig. 3B) and the protein content of α-SMA (Fig. 3C) were at least 2-fold higher in null livers relative to controls under both feeding conditions. This was mediated by the activation of the canonical TGFβ-Smad2/3 pathway, as indicated by increased Smad2/3 phosphorylation (Fig. 3C) and by the ~3-to-4–fold decrease in the mRNA (Table S3-S4) and protein (Fig. 3C) levels of TGFβ-Smad2/3 inhibitor, Smad7, arising from elevated plasma and hepatic TNF□ levels [35]. Liver-specific rescuing of CEACAM1 reversed the pro-fibrogenic effect of global *Ceacam1* null deletion even when mice were fed a HF diet (Fig. 3A), and this was mediated by inactivating the TGFβ-Smad2/3 pathway [as marked by blunted Smad2/3 phosphorylation (Fig. 3C) and restoring hepatic Smad7 mRNA (Table S3-S4) and protein levels (Fig. 3C) in response to normalizing TNFα levels].

As previously reported [36], global *Ceacam1* null mutation caused an increase in plasma endothelin-1 (Et-1) levels by 2-to-4–fold irrespective of the diet (Table 2), likely in response to hyperinsulinemia [37], as evidenced by its reversal in the normoinsulinemic *Cc1*$^{-/-xliver+}$ mice (Table 2). Plasma ET-1 levels (Table 2) as well as its hepatic mRNA levels and that of its receptor A (*Etar*) that mediates its pro-fibrogenic activity (Fig. 3B) were elevated in *Cc1*$^{-/-}$ but not *Cc1*$^{-/-xliver+}$ liver-rescue mice. Mechanistically, this could stem from activation of NF-κB which, in the presence of low NO levels and oxidative stress, could also induce the transcription of the pro-fibrogenic platelet-derived growth factor-B (PDGF-B) either directly or indirectly via activating HIF-1α [38, 39], as manifested by their higher hepatic mRNA levels in null mice (Fig. 3B). Liver-specific rescuing of CEACAM1 normalized plasma (Table 2) and hepatic mRNA levels of ET-1 and PDGF-B (Fig. 3B) via inactivating NF-kB and HIF-1α pathways in the normoinsulinemic (Fig. 2C-3C) and normoglycemic *Cc1*$^{-/-xliver+}$ mice.

HF feeding for 5 months caused similar molecular and histopathologic anomalies to those caused by 3 months of high-fat intake. Pertinent analyses are summarized through evaluating NAFLD activity score (NAS) per NIH guidelines (Table 3). As shown, RD-fed

*Cc1*$^{-/-}$ mice did not exhibit the full spectrum of NASH even at 8 months of age (NAS<4). In contrast, fed a HF diet for 5 months, *Cc1*$^{-/-}$ mice developed NASH at a NAS score of >7 (Table 3). Liver-specific rescuing of *Ceacam1* reversed the NAS score to <4 even after 5 months of HF intake and protected against NASH (Table 3).

**Discussion**

Despite prevailing controversy regarding the role of insulin resistance in the pathogenesis of NASH, it has been accepted that insulin resistance underlies the switch from simple steatosis to NAFLD [119, 120]. Furthermore, the progression from steatohepatitis to NASH implicates a myriad of molecular and cellular events including oxidative stress, nitroso-redox imbalance, apoptosis, hepatocellular injury and chicken-wire fibrosis. The metabolic and histopathological phenotypes of *Cc1*$^{-/-}$ [132] and L-SACC1 liver-specific inactive mice [89] have provided an *in vivo* demonstration of this paradigm of NASH pathogenesis. Global and liver-specific null deletion or inactivation of *Ceacam1* impaired insulin clearance to cause chronic hyperinsulinemia that led to insulin resistance, hepatic steatosis and visceral obesity [64]. Consistent with elevated pro-inflammatory response to steatosis, *Ceacam1* mutants developed steatohepatitis in the presence of normal cholesterol homeostasis when fed a regular diet [89, 130, 133].

Together with the reversal of the metabolic dysregulation in *Cc1*$^{-/-}$ mice by liver-specific reconstitution of CEACAM1 [90], this assigned a key role for impaired insulin clearance-driven hyperinsulinemia in the switch from simple hepatic steatosis to NAFLD. In support of the well-documented role of inflammation in initiating hepatocellular injury [149], and of the regulatory role of CEACAM1 at the juncture of metabolic and immune regulation of liver function [134], *Ceacam1* mutant livers also developed low-grade fibrosis that progressed into more severe fibrosis in response to high-fat feeding [89, 132]. This pointed at a potentially key role for altered hepatic CEACAM1-dependent pathways in NASH progression. The current studies demonstrated that liver-specific reconstitution of CEACAM1 prevented the development and the progression of hepatic fibrosis together with other key features of NASH in global $Cc1^{-/-}$ nulls after prolonged period of high-fat intake. This provides an *in vivo* manifest of how the loss of hepatic CEACAM1 regulates, not only the switch from simple steatosis to NAFLD, but also the escalation to NASH, including the development of advanced fibrosis and apoptosis.

As in L-SACC1 mutants [89], HF diet induced lipid peroxidation in $Cc1^{-/-}$ but not wild-type mice. This nitroso-redox imbalance caused by high-fat diet could initiate peroxidative events commonly associated with necrotic damage and apoptosis in null livers [113, 150]. This could be triggered at least in part, by inducing hepatic TNFα [151] and amplifying its cytotoxic effect through the compromised GSH-based mitochondrial defense system associated with lower NPC1 and possible partitioning of free cholesterol to mitochondria in null mice [150], as was shown for L-SACC1 mice [89]. Reversal of this phenotype in null mice by reintroducing CEACAM1 specifically to the liver further underscored the role of the loss of CEACAM1 in the pathogenesis of oxidative stress and inflammation commonly implicated in NASH [115, 118, 136].

Fibrosis in $Cc1^{-/-}$ mice was mediated by activated TGFβ-Smad2/3 canonical pathways. This was driven by increased production of ET-1 and PDGF-B, two key pro-fibrogenic effectors. Increased levels of ET-1 and its *ETar* receptors that mediate its fibrogenic activities could be partly driven by hyperinsulinemia [146], as demonstrated by normalization of their levels upon redelivery of *Ceacam1* to the liver and recovering normoinsulinemia and insulin sensitivity in $Cc1^{-/-\text{xliver}+}$ mice. As previously shown, the vascular endothelium of $Cc1^{-/-}$ mice exhibited repression of Akt-eNOS-dependent NO synthesis pathways, resulting from hyperinsulinemia-driven reduction in insulin receptors [145]. The increase in ET-1 in the presence of low NO and oxidative stress, could result from activation of NF-κB directly or indirectly via HIF-1α [147]. This could tip the vasomotor balance towards vasoconstriction that could in turn, activate hepatic stellate cells to cause fibrosis [152].

Activated NF-κB could also induce the transcription of PDGF-B directly and in corporation with HIF-1α [147, 148]. Consistent with PKC inducing PDGF-B expression under fasting hyperglycemic conditions [153], HF activated PKC-ζ in $Cc1^{-/-}$, but not wild-type mice in parallel to increasing their lipid peroxidation. Elevated PDGF-B could synergize with ET-1 to induce collagen production by triggering proliferation of hepatic stellate cells [152]. Normalizing ET-1 and PDGF-B by curbing inflammation and oxidative stress in mice with liver-specific redelivery of CEACAM1 prevented hepatic fibrosis. Reversal of NASH in $Cc1^{-/-}$ upon restoring their hepatic CEACAM1 expression emphasized the key role of hepatic CEACAM1 in maintaining normal liver architecture and function.

*Strengths and weaknesses*

The gain-of-function model used in the current studies identified CEACAM1 as a defense system against hepatic fibrosis. In support of these findings, liver grafts with low

CEACAM1 manifested an increase in ischemia-reperfusion injury inflammation and decreased function in wild-type recipient mice and caused post-reperfusion damage in liver transplant human recipients [154]. Interestingly, PPARγ and GLP-1 receptor agonists that have are used to treat insulin-resistant NAFLD patients [121, 122] with advanced fibrosis [155] induce Ceacam1 transcription [156]. Thus, it is likely that the effectiveness of these drugs is mediated at least in part, by their positive effect on CEACAM1 expression and function. Our studies promote elevation of hepatic CEACAM1 expression as an efficacious targeted therapeutical approach not only to curb insulin resistance and NAFLD, but also to prevent or reverse fibrosis without causing the body weight gain often observed in patients treated with PPARγ agonists. Thus, drug development followed by clinical studies are needed to test whether therapeutic targeting of CEACAM1 constitutes a more effective approach against fibrosis.

*Conclusions*

The current studies demonstrated that liver-specific reconstitution of CEACAM1 in $Ccl^{-/-}$ nulls reversed hyperinsulinemia-driven metabolic and histopathological features of NASH and prevented the development of fibrosis and liver dysfunction. We propose that targeting CEACAM1 could be a novel therapeutic approach against NASH and its escalation to end-stage liver disease.

**Figure Legends**

Fig. 1. Hepatic expression of the transgene and metabolic analysis of 6-month-old mice. 3-month-old male mice were fed RD or HF diet for 3 months (n>5 per genotype/feeding group). (A) CEACAM1 protein level was analyzed by immunoblotting (Ib) liver lysates with polyclonal antibodies against mouse (mCC1) or rat (rCC1) CEACAM1 (upper gels). To normalize for protein loading, the lower half of the membrane was immunoblotted with α-Tubulin. Gels represent 2 experiments performed on 2 different mice/genotype. (B) mice were subjected to an intraperitoneal injection of insulin (0.75 U/kg BW) (panels *i, iii*), and glucose (1.5 g/kg BW) (panels *ii* and *iv*) to evaluate blood glucose levels at 0-180- or 0-120-min post-injection, respectively.

Fig. 2. Histological and biochemical analysis of RD or HF-fed mice. Livers of 6-month-old mice (n=5/genotype) were extracted and sectioned for (A) H&E staining to detect inflammatory foci (blue arrows) and microvesicular lipid droplets. (B) Hepatic fatty acid synthase activity (panel *i*) and hepatic palmitate oxidation (panel *ii*) were assayed in overnight fasted mice. Assays were performed in triplicate (n>5). Values are expressed as means ± SEM. $^{a}P\leq0.05$ vs $Ccl^{+/+}$; $^{b}P\leq0.05$ vs L-CC1; and $^{c}P\leq0.05$ vs $Ccl^{-/-}$. (C) Western blot analysis was performed on liver lysates by immunoblotting (Ib) with antibodies against phosphorylated signaling proteins (α-pNF-κB, α-pStat3, α-peNOS, α-pPKCζ) normalized against their non-phosphorylated counterparts immunodetected on parallel gels. (D) Tunnel staining on liver sections to detect apoptotic bodies. CHOP protein was detected by immunoblotting with α-CHOP antibody normalized against total protein ($\alpha$-tubulin) loaded on parallel gel. Gels represent more than 2 experiments performed on different mice/genotype.

Fig. 3. Histological analysis of RD or HF-fed mice. (A) Sirius red staining to detect interstitial collagen deposition in the parenchyma of $Cc1^{-/-}$ mice – Panel *iii*. Representative images are shown. Fibrosis scoring was evaluated by Brunt criteria in the accompanying table. (B) mRNA analysis of fibrotic markers in liver tissue of RD or HF-fed mice normalized to Gapdh or 18S respectively. Values are expressed as means $\pm$ SEM. [a]$P \leq 0.05$ vs $Cc1^{+/+}$; [b]$P \leq 0.05$ vs L-CC1; and [c]$P \leq 0.05$ vs $Cc1^{-/-}$. (C) Western blot analysis was performed on liver lysates by immunoblotting (Ib) with antibodies against phosphorylated signaling proteins ($\alpha$-pSmad2, $\alpha$-pSmad3) normalized against their non-phosphorylated counterparts immunodetected on parallel gels. Smad7 and SMA proteins was detected by immunoblotting with $\alpha$-Smad7 or $\alpha$-SMA antibodies normalized against total proteins ($\alpha$-tubulin) loaded on parallel gels. Gels represent more than 2 experiments performed on different mice/genotype.

Fig. S1: PCR genotyping of mice. Liver lysates from 6-month-old mice were subjected to PCR analysis using primers listed in the table at the bottom of the illustration. Apolipoprotein A1 promoter was used to drive forced liver-specific expression of rat *Ceacam1* gene in L-CC1 mice followed by their crossbreeding with global null mice ($Cc1^{-/-}$) to generate four littermates with wild-type ($Cc1^{+/+}$), null $Cc1^{-/-}$ and L-CC1 as controls, and $Cc1^{-/-xliver+}$ as liver-specific Ceacam1 rescue mice. The null allele in $Cc1^{-/-}$ and $Cc1^{-/-xliver+}$ was detected at 750bp, the transgenic rat Ceacam1 of

LCC-1 and $Ccl^{-/-\text{xliver+}}$ was detected at 650bp, and wild-type endogenous mouse allele in

$Ccl^{+/+}$ or L-CC1 was detected at 250bp.

**References**

[1]     Buzzetti E, Pinzani M, Tsochatzis EA. The multiple-hit pathogenesis of non-alcoholic fatty liver disease (NAFLD). Metabolism. 2016;65:1038-48.

[2]     Younossi ZM. Non-alcoholic fatty liver disease - A global public health perspective. J Hepatol. 2019;70:531-44.

[3]     Tilg H, Moschen AR. Evolution of inflammation in nonalcoholic fatty liver disease: the multiple parallel hits hypothesis. Hepatology. 2010;52:1836-46.

[4]     Gan LT, Van Rooyen DM, Koina ME, McCuskey RS, Teoh NC, Farrell GC. Hepatocyte free cholesterol lipotoxicity results from JNK1-mediated mitochondrial injury and is HMGB1 and TLR4-dependent. J Hepatol. 2014;61:1376-84.

[5]     Fuchs M, Sanyal AJ. Lipotoxicity in NASH. J Hepatol. 2012;56:291-3.

[6]     Dallio M, Sangineto M, Romeo M, Villani R, Romano AD, Loguercio C, et al. Immunity as Cornerstone of Non-Alcoholic Fatty Liver Disease: The Contribution of Oxidative Stress in the Disease Progression. Int J Mol Sci. 2021;22.

[7]     Masarone M, Rosato V, Dallio M, Gravina AG, Aglitti A, Loguercio C, et al. Role of Oxidative Stress in Pathophysiology of Nonalcoholic Fatty Liver Disease. Oxidative medicine and cellular longevity. 2018;2018:9547613.

[8]     Thomas DD, Corkey BE, Istfan NW, Apovian CM. Hyperinsulinemia: An Early Indicator of Metabolic Dysfunction. J Endocr Soc. 2019;3:1727-47.

[9]     Gastaldelli A, Cusi K. From NASH to diabetes and from diabetes to NASH: Mechanisms and treatment options. JHEP Rep. 2019;1:312-28.

[10]    Stefan N, Haring HU, Cusi K. Non-alcoholic fatty liver disease: causes, diagnosis, cardiometabolic consequences, and treatment strategies. Lancet Diabetes Endocrinol. 2019;7:313-24.

[11]    Bril F, Lomonaco R, Orsak B, Ortiz-Lopez C, Webb A, Tio F, et al. Relationship between disease severity, hyperinsulinemia, and impaired insulin clearance in patients with nonalcoholic steatohepatitis. Hepatology. 2014;59:2178-87.

[12]    Heinrich G, Muturi HT, Rezaei K, Al-Share QY, DeAngelis AM, Bowman TA, et al. Reduced hepatic carcinoembryonic antigen-related cell adhesion molecule 1 level in obesity. Front Endocrinol (Lausanne). 2017;8:54.

[13]    Lee W. The CEACAM1 expression is decreased in the liver of severely obese patients with or without diabetes. Diagn Pathol. 2011;6:40.

[14]    Najjar SM, Perdomo G. Hepatic Insulin Clearance: Mechanism and Physiology. Physiology (Bethesda). 2019;34:198-215.

[15]    Xu E, Dubois MJ, Leung N, Charbonneau A, Turbide C, Avramoglu RK, et al. Targeted disruption of carcinoembryonic antigen-related cell adhesion molecule 1 promotes diet-induced hepatic steatosis and insulin resistance. Endocrinology. 2009;150:3503-12.

[16]    DeAngelis AM, Heinrich G, Dai T, Bowman TA, Patel PR, Lee SJ, et al. Carcinoembryonic antigen-related cell adhesion molecule 1: a link between insulin and lipid metabolism. Diabetes. 2008;57:2296-303.

[17]    Ghadieh HE, Russo L, Muturi HT, Ghanem SS, Manaserh IH, Noh HL, et al. Hyperinsulinemia drives hepatic insulin resistance in male mice with liver-specific Ceacam1 deletion independently of lipolysis. Metabolism. 2019;93:33-43.

[18]    Poy MN, Yang Y, Rezaei K, Fernstrom MA, Lee AD, Kido Y, et al. CEACAM1 regulates insulin clearance in liver. Nat Genet. 2002;30:270-6.

[19]    Najjar SM, Yang Y, Fernstrom MA, Lee SJ, Deangelis AM, Rjaily GA, et al. Insulin acutely decreases hepatic fatty acid synthase activity. Cell Metab. 2005;2:43-53.

[20]    Najjar SM, Russo L. CEACAM1 loss links inflammation to insulin resistance in obesity and non-alcoholic steatohepatitis (NASH). Semin Immunopathol. 2014;36:55-71.

[21]    Najjar SM, Ledford KJ, Abdallah SL, Paus A, Russo L, Kaw MK, et al. Ceacam1 deletion causes vascular alterations in large vessels. Am J Physiol Endocrinol Metab. 2013;305:E519-29.

[22]    Ghosh S, Kaw M, Patel PR, Ledford KJ, Bowman TA, McLnerney MF, et al. Mice with null mutation of Ceacam I develop nonalcoholic steatohepatitis. Hepat Med: Res Evidence. 2010;2010:69-78.

[23]    Ghadieh HE, Abu Helal R, Muturi HT, Issa DD, Russo L, Abdallah SL, et al. Loss of Hepatic Carcinoembryonic Antigen-Related Cell Adhesion Molecule 1 Links Nonalcoholic Steatohepatitis to Atherosclerosis. Hepatol Commun. 2020;4:1591-609.

[24]     Horst AK, Najjar SM, Wagener C, Tiegs G. CEACAM1 in Liver Injury,

Metabolic and Immune Regulation. Int J Mol Sci. 2018;19.

[25]     Russo L, Muturi HT, Ghadieh HE, Ghanem SS, Bowman TA, Noh HL, et al.

Liver-specific reconstitution of CEACAM1 reverses the metabolic abnormalities

caused by its global deletion in male mice. Diabetologia. 2017;60:2463-74.

[26]     Al-Share QY, DeAngelis AM, Lester SG, Bowman TA, Ramakrishnan SK,

Abdallah SL, et al. Forced Hepatic Overexpression of CEACAM1 Curtails Diet-

Induced Insulin Resistance. Diabetes. 2015;64:2780-90.

[27]     Tacke F, Zimmermann HW. Macrophage heterogeneity in liver injury and

fibrosis. J Hepatol. 2014;60:1090-6.

[28]     Adelaja A, Hoffmann A. Signaling Crosstalk Mechanisms That May Fine-Tune

Pathogen-Responsive NFkappaB. Front Immunol. 2019;10:433.

[29]     Suryavanshi SV, Kulkarni YA. NF-kappabeta: A Potential Target in the

Management of Vascular Complications of Diabetes. Front Pharmacol.

2017;8:798.

[30]     Gregor MF, Hotamisligil GS. Inflammatory mechanisms in obesity. Ann Rev

Immunol. 2011;29:415-45.

[31]     Abdel-Razzak Z, Garlatti M, Aggerbeck M, Barouki R. Determination of

interleukin-4-responsive region in the human cytochrome P450 2E1 gene

promoter. Biochem, Pharmacol,. 2004;68:1371-81.

[32]    Mari M, Caballero F, Colell A, Morales A, Caballeria J, Fernandez A, et al. Mitochondrial free cholesterol loading sensitizes to TNF- and Fas-mediated steatohepatitis. Cell Metab. 2006;4:185-98.

[33]    Cai D, Yuan M, Frantz DF, Melendez PA, Hansen L, Lee J, et al. Local and systemic insulin resistance resulting from hepatic activation of IKK-beta and NF-kappaB. Nat Med. 2005;11:183-90.

[34]    Manicassamy S, Gupta S, Huang Z, Sun Z. Protein kinase C-theta-mediated signals enhance CD4+ T cell survival by up-regulating Bcl-xL. J Immunol. 2006;176:6709-16.

[35]    Nagarajan RP, Chen F, Li W, Vig E, Harrington MA, Nakshatri H, et al. Repression of transforming-growth-factor-beta-mediated transcription by nuclear factor kappaB. Biochem J. 2000;348 Pt 3:591-6.

[36]    Russo L, Muturi HT, Ghadieh HE, Wisniewski AM, Morgan EE, Quadri SS, et al. Liver-specific rescuing of CEACAM1 reverses endothelial and cardiovascular abnormalities in male mice with null deletion of Ceacam1 gene. Mol Metab. 2018;9:98-113.

[37]    Mahmoud AM, Szczurek MR, Blackburn BK, Mey JT, Chen Z, Robinson AT, et al. Hyperinsulinemia augments endothelin-1 protein expression and impairs vasodilation of human skeletal muscle arterioles. Physiol Rep. 2016;4.

[38]    van Uden P, Kenneth NS, Rocha S. Regulation of hypoxia-inducible factor-1alpha by NF-kappaB. Biochem J. 2008;412:477-84.

[39] Au PY, Martin N, Chau H, Moemeni B, Chia M, Liu FF, et al. The oncogene PDGF-B provides a key switch from cell death to survival induced by TNF. Oncogene. 2005;24:3196-205.

[40] Lee SJ, Heinrich G, Fedorova L, Al-Share QY, Ledford KJ, Fernstrom MA, et al. Development of nonalcoholic steatohepatitis in insulin-resistant liver-specific S503A carcinoembryonic antigen-related cell adhesion molecule 1 mutant mice. Gastroenterology. 2008;135:2084-95.

[41] Wan J, Weiss E, Ben Mkaddem S, Mabire M, Choinier PM, Thibault-Sogorb T, et al. LC3-associated phagocytosis in myeloid cells, a fireman that restrains inflammation and liver fibrosis, via immunoreceptor inhibitory signaling. Autophagy. 2020;16:1526-8.

[42] Musso G, Gambino R, Cassader M. Cholesterol metabolism and the pathogenesis of non-alcoholic steatohepatitis. Prog Lipid Res. 2013;52:175-91.

[43] Carter-Kent C, Zein NN, Feldstein AE. Cytokines in the pathogenesis of fatty liver and disease progression to steatohepatitis: implications for treatment. Am J Gastroenterol. 2008;103:1036-42.

[44] Friedman SL. Mechanisms of hepatic fibrogenesis. Gastroenterology. 2008;134:1655-69.

[45] Yokota T, Ma RC, Park JY, Isshiki K, Sotiropoulos KB, Rauniyar RK, et al. Role of protein kinase C on the expression of platelet-derived growth factor and endothelin-1 in the retina of diabetic rats and cultured retinal capillary pericytes. Diabetes. 2003;52:838-45.

[46]    Nakamura K, Kageyama S, Kaldas FM, Hirao H, Ito T, Kadono K, et al. Hepatic

CEACAM1 expression indicates donor liver quality and prevents early

transplantation injury. J Clin Invest. 2020;130:2689-704.

[47]    Musso G, Cassader M, Paschetta E, Gambino R. Pioglitazone for advanced

fibrosis in nonalcoholic steatohepatitis: New evidence, new challenges.

Hepatology. 2017;65:1058-61.

[48]    Ghadieh HE, Muturi HT, Russo L, Marino CC, Ghanem SS, Khuder SS, et al.

Exenatide induces carcinoembryonic antigen-related cell adhesion molecule 1

expression to prevent hepatic steatosis. Hepatol Commun. 2018;2:35-47.

**Tables and Figures**

**Table 1: Plasma and Tissue Metabolic Parameters**

|  | $Ccl^{+/+}$ | L-CC1 | $Ccl^{-/-}$ | $Ccl^{-/-xliver+}$ |
|---|---|---|---|---|
| **a) RD** | | | | |
| % Fat mass | $12.6 \pm 0.6$ | $11.3 \pm 0.4$ | $17.2 \pm 0.6^{ab}$ | $13.1 \pm 0.1^{c}$ |
| % Lean mass | $72.5 \pm 1.0$ | $77.0 \pm 2.1$ | $63.7 \pm 1.0^{ab}$ | $73.1 \pm 1.3^{c}$ |
| Plasma NEFA (mEq/l) | $0.5 \pm 0.0$ | $0.5 \pm 0.1$ | $1.0 \pm 0.1^{ab}$ | $0.4 \pm 0.2^{c}$ |
| Plasma Insulin (pM) | $76.6 \pm 1.2$ | $74.4 \pm 1.0$ | $140.6 \pm 5.1^{ab}$ | $74.1 \pm 0.8^{c}$ |
| Plasma C-peptide (pM) | $433.7 \pm 1.9$ | $415.8 \pm 11.6$ | $583.7 \pm 3.1^{ab}$ | $431.6 \pm 0.4^{c}$ |
| C-peptide/Insulin | $5.7 \pm 0.1$ | $5.6 \pm 0.2$ | $4.0 \pm 0.1^{ab}$ | $5.8 \pm 0.1^{c}$ |
| Fasting blood glucose (mg/dl) | $95 \pm 8$ | $75 \pm 7$ | $89 \pm 2$ | $73 \pm 8$ |
| Fed blood glucose (mg/dl) | $104 \pm 9$ | $93 \pm 5$ | $152 \pm 7^{ab}$ | $85 \pm 5^{c}$ |
| Hepatic triglycerides (µg/mg) | $59.1 \pm 4.3$ | $57.8 \pm 1.1$ | $84.1 \pm 7.1^{ab}$ | $57.9 \pm 6.1^{c}$ |
| Plasma triglycerides (mg/dl) | $51.4 \pm 0.7$ | $50.7 \pm 2.1$ | $51.9 \pm 0.8$ | $49.9 \pm 1.1$ |
| Hepatic total cholesterol (mg/dl) | $71 \pm 6.1$ | $75.7 \pm 3.9$ | $75.3 \pm 3.4$ | $75.3 \pm 3.4$ |
| **b) HF** | | | | |
| % Fat mass | $25.4 \pm 0.6$ | $26.9 \pm 0.4$ | $30.6 \pm 0.5^{ab}$ | $24.5 \pm 1.1^{c}$ |
| % Lean mass | $59.5 \pm 0.7$ | $59.5 \pm 1.0$ | $54.1 \pm 0.6^{ab}$ | $62. \pm 1.0^{c}$ |
| Plasma NEFA (mEq/l) | $0.6 \pm 0.2$ | $0.6 \pm 0.1$ | $1.3 \pm 0.1^{ab}$ | $0.5 \pm 0.2^{c}$ |
| Plasma Insulin (pM) | $107.3 \pm 5.9$ | $104.4 \pm 10.6$ | $210.4 \pm 3.8^{ab}$ | $94.7 \pm 2.2^{c}$ |
| Plasma C-peptide (pM) | $697 \pm 20$ | $702 \pm 11$ | $1065 \pm 32^{ab}$ | $690 \pm 2^{c}$ |
| C-peptide/Insulin | $6.9 \pm 0.6$ | $7.4 \pm 0.3$ | $4.9 \pm 0.2^{ab}$ | $7.3 \pm 0.2^{c}$ |
| Fasting blood glucose (mg/dl) | $116 \pm 6$ | $120 \pm 9$ | $157 \pm 7^{ab}$ | $120 \pm 5^{c}$ |
| Fed blood glucose (mg/dl) | $116 \pm 1$ | $122 \pm 8$ | $171 \pm 5^{ab}$ | $114 \pm 1^{c}$ |
| Hepatic triglycerides (µg/mg) | $95 \pm 4$ | $76 \pm 6$ | $170 \pm 31^{ab}$ | $82 \pm 4^{c}$ |
| Plasma triglycerides (mg/dl) | $52.2 \pm 0.9$ | $47.7 \pm 1.2$ | $45.7 \pm 0.9$ | $43.7 \pm 2.7$ |
| Hepatic total cholesterol (mg/dl) | $81.2 \pm 4.0$ | $82.4 \pm 2.5$ | $84 \pm 2.8$ | $79.2 \pm 4.4$ |

Male mice were fed a HF or kept on RD diet for 3 months starting at 3 months of age ($n \geq 5$-8 mice/genotype/feeding group). Retro-orbital blood and tissues were collected at 11:00 a.m. following an overnight fast. Steady-state-C-peptide/insulin was calculated as a measure of insulin clearance. Values are expressed as mean±SEM. $^{a}P<0.05$ vs $Ccl^{+/+}$, $^{b}P<0.05$ vs L-CC1, $^{c}P<0.05$ vs $Ccl^{-/-}$.

**Table 2: Plasma and Tissue Biochemistry**

|  | $Ccl^{+/+}$ | L-CC1 | $Ccl^{-/-}$ | $Ccl^{-/-xliver+}$ |
|---|---|---|---|---|
| **a)  RD** | | | | |
| Plasma TNFα (pg/ml) | $4.6 \pm 0.2$ | $4.7 \pm 0.2$ | $9.0 \pm 0.1\,^{ab}$ | $4.5 \pm 0.3\,^{c}$ |
| Plasma IL-6 (pg/ml) | $34.6 \pm 1.4$ | $34.0 \pm 0.7$ | $57.1 \pm 2.1\,^{ab}$ | $33.8 \pm 1.0\,^{c}$ |
| Plasma AST (mU/ml) | $44.7 \pm 5.2$ | $36.7 \pm 6.4$ | $87.7 \pm 5.0\,^{ab}$ | $48.9 \pm 7.5\,^{c}$ |
| Plasma ALT (mU/ml) | $7.7 \pm 1.2$ | $8.2 \pm 1.0$ | $14.8 \pm 0.5\,^{ab}$ | $9.3 \pm 1.5\,^{c}$ |
| Hepatic NO (μM/μgx10$^{-1}$) | $4.0 \pm 0.0$ | $4.0 \pm 0.0$ | $2.0 \pm 0.0\,^{ab}$ | $3.0 \pm 0.0\,^{c}$ |
| Hepatic GSH (μmol/g wt) | $1.8 \pm 0.1$ | $1.8 \pm 0.0$ | $1.8 \pm 0.0$ | $1.7 \pm 0.0$ |
| Plasma ET-1 (pg/ml) | $4.2 \pm 0.4$ | $3.6 \pm 0.8$ | $11.7 \pm 0.4\,^{ab}$ | $4.6 \pm 0.5\,^{c}$ |
| **b)  HF** | | | | |
| Plasma TNFα (pg/ml) | $5.0 \pm 0.2$ | $5.5 \pm 0.4$ | $9.7 \pm 0.3\,^{ab}$ | $4.9 \pm 0.2\,^{c}$ |
| Plasma IL-6 (pg/ml) | $40.3 \pm 1.3$ | $39.8 \pm 3.2$ | $63.7 \pm 1.7\,^{ab}$ | $36.0 \pm 2.5\,^{c}$ |
| Plasma AST (mU/ml) | $77.6 \pm 8.2$ | $70.2 \pm 9.6$ | $136 \pm 17\,^{ab}$ | $58.9 \pm 10.1\,^{c}$ |
| Plasma ALT (mU/ml) | $16.8 \pm 2.4$ | $15.1 \pm 1.6$ | $27.0 \pm 2.5\,^{ab}$ | $13.4 \pm 2.5\,^{c}$ |
| Hepatic NO (μM/μgx10$^{-1}$) | $5.0 \pm 0.0$ | $4.0 \pm 0.0$ | $2.0 \pm 0.0\,^{ab}$ | $5.0 \pm 0.0\,^{c}$ |
| Hepatic GSH (μmol/g wt) | $4.3 \pm 0.2$ | $4.3 \pm 0.2$ | $1.6 \pm 0.0\,^{ab}$ | $4.3 \pm 0.2\,^{c}$ |
| Plasma ET-1 (pg/ml) | $15.6 \pm 2.1$ | $15.2 \pm 2.4$ | $33.7 \pm 3.4\,^{ab}$ | $13.6 \pm 3.6\,^{c}$ |

Male mice were fed a HF or kept on RD diet for 3 months starting at 3 months of age (n≥5-8 mice/genotype/feeding group). Retro-orbital blood and tissues were collected at 11:00 a.m. following an overnight fast. Values are expressed as mean±SEM. *$^{a}P<0.05$ vs $Ccl^{+/+}$, $^{b}P<0.05$ vs L-CC1, $^{c}P<0.05$ vs $Ccl^{-/-}$.*

**Table 3: NAFLD Activity Score (NAS)**

| Group | Diet | Mice/ number | Steatosis | Inflammation | | Ballooning | Total NAS | NASH |
| | | | Micro/ macro (0-3) | Lobular (0-3) | Portal (0-3) | Hepatocyte (0-2) | Score (0-8) | |
|---|---|---|---|---|---|---|---|---|
| $Ccl^{+/+}$ | RD | >3 | 0 | $\leq 1$ | 0 | 0 | $\leq 1$ | No |
| $Ccl^{+/+}$ | HF | >3 | 2 | $\leq 2$ | 0 | 0 | $\leq 4$ | No |
| L-CC1 | RD | >4 | 0 | $\leq 1$ | 0 | 0 | $\leq 1$ | No |
| L-CC1 | HF | >3 | 2 | $\leq 2$ | 0 | 0 | $\leq 4$ | No |
| $Ccl^{-/-}$ | RD | >3 | $\leq 2$ | 1 | $\leq 1$ | 0 | $\leq 4$ | No |
| $Ccl^{-/-}$ | HF | >3 | 3 | 2 | $\leq 2$ | 0 | $\leq 7$ | YES |
| $Ccl^{-/-}_{xliver+}$ | RD | >3 | 0 | $\leq 1$ | 0 | 0 | $\leq 1$ | No |
| $Ccl^{-/-}_{xliver+}$ | HF | >3 | 2 | $\leq 2$ | 0 | 0 | $\leq 4$ | No |

Male mice were fed a HF or kept on RD diet for 5 months starting at 3 months of age (n≥3-6 mice/genotype/feeding group). NAS score was evaluated based on NIH guidelines.

**Table S1: qRT-PCR Analysis of Ceacam1 mRNA Levels**

|  |  | $Cc1^{+/+}$ | L-CC1 | $Cc1^{-/-}$ | $Cc1^{-/-xliver+}$ |
|---|---|---|---|---|---|
| **Liver** |  |  |  |  |  |
|  | *mCc1* | 2.4 ± 0.8 | 1.7±0.5 | Negl. | Negl. |
|  | *rCc1* | Negl. | 5.4±0.1 | Negl. | 5.4 ± 0.2 |
| **Hypothalamus** |  |  |  |  |  |
|  | *mCc1* | 1.4 ± 0.3 | 1.1 ± 0.1 | Negl. | Negl. |
|  | *rCc1* | Negl. | Negl. | Negl | Negl. |
| **WAT** |  |  |  |  |  |
|  | *mCc1* | 1.6 ± 0.2 | 1.5 ± 0.1 | Negl. | Negl. |
|  | *rCc1* | Negl. | Negl. | Negl | Negl. |
| **Skeletal Muscle** |  |  |  |  |  |
|  | *mCc1* | 0.9 ± 0.1 | 0.8 ± 0.1 | Negl. | Negl. |
|  | *rCc1* | Negl. | Negl. | Negl | Negl. |

Tissues were removed from overnight fasted 6-month-old male mice (n ≥ 5 mice/genotype) to analyze mRNA by qRT-PCR (normalized to Gapdh or 36B4). Values are expressed as mean ± SEM. Negl., negligible

**Table S2: Gene-Specific Primer Sequences**

| Primer | Forward Sequence (5'-3') | Reverse Sequence (5'-3') |
|---|---|---|
| *α-Sma* | CGTGGCTATTCCTTCGTTAC | TGCCAGGAGACTCCATCC |
| Bcl2 | GTGGTGGAGGAACTCTTCAG | GTTCCACAAAGGCATCCCAG |
| *Cd4* | TCACCTGGAAGTTCTCTGACC | GGAATCAAAACGATCAAACTGCG |
| *Cd8* | CTCTGGCTGGTCTTCAGTATGA | TCTTTGCCGTATGGTTGGTTT |
| *Cd11b* | TACGTAATTGGGGTGGGAA | GTGCCCTCAATTGCAAAGAT |
| *Cd36* | TCTTGGCTACAGCAAGGCGACATA | AGCTATGCAGCATGGAACATGACG |
| *Cd68* | CCTCGCCCTAGTCCAAGGTC | CGATTCGGATTTGAATTTGGGCT |
| Chop | CCACCACACCTGAAAGCAGAA | AGGTGCCCCCAATTTCATCT |
| *Ctgf* | AATGTCAGTGCGCAGCCGAAGCA | AGGGGTCACGCTCCGTACACAG |
| *Col6α3* | GTCAGCTGAGTCTTGTGCTGT | ACCTAGAGAACGTTACCTCACT |
| Cyp2E1 | CCATCGGCACCATGGCGGTT | GCCCGAAGCGCTTTGCCAAC |
| *Elastase* | GTTGGGCACAAACAGACC | GCAAACTCAGCCACAGG |
| *Et-1* | GGTGGAAGGAAGGAAACTAC | CAAGAAGAGGCAGAAAGGCA |
| *Etar* | AACAAGTGTATGAGGACGGC | GGCCAAGATGAAGGAAAGAA |
| *Etbr* | CAGTCTTCTGCCTGGTCCTC | GGACTGCTTTTCCTCAAACG |
| *Fasn* | ACTGTGAGAAGCATGTCCCTGGAA | AAGCAACCTCCACTCCTCTGCTTA |
| Fatp1 | GCAGAAGACGCAGGAAGA | GGACGTGGCTGTGTATGG |
| Foxp3 | CCCAGGAAAGACAGCAACCTT | TTTCACAACCAGGCCACTTG |
| *F4/80* | CAAGGAGGACAGAGTTTATCGTG | CTTTGGCTATGGGCTTCCAGTC |
| *Gapdh* | CCAGGTTGTCTCCTGCGACT | ATACCAGGAAATGAGCTTGACAAAGT |
| *Gr1* | GATGGATTTTGCGTTGCTCT | CAGAGTAGTGGGGCAGATG |
| *HGF* | CTTCTCCTTGGCCTTGAATG | CCTGACACCACTTGGGAGTA |

| *Hif1α* | TCCATGTGACCATGAGGAAA | CTTCCACGTTGCTGACTTGA |
|---|---|---|
| *IL-1β* | CCCTGCAGCTGGAGAGTGTGG | TATTCTGTCCATTGAGGTGGAG |
| *IL-4* | AGGTCACAGGAGAAGGGACGCC | TGCGAAGCACCTTGGAAGCCC |
| *IL-6* | CTTGGGACTGCCGCTGGTGA | TGCAAGTGCATCATCGTTGT |
| *IL-10* | CACAAAGCAGCCTTGCAGAA | AGAGCAGGCAGCATAGCAGTG |
| *IL-13* | TGTTTCGCCACGGCCCCTTC | TGCTCAAGCTGCTGCCTGCC |
| *Irf8* | CGTGGAAGACGAGGTTACGCTG | GCTGAATGGTGTGTGTCATAGGC |
| *Ifnγ* | ATGAACGCTACACACTGCATC | CCATCCTTTTGCCAGTTCCTC |
| *mCc1* | AATCTGCCCCTGGCGCTTGGAGCC | AAATCGCACAGTCGCCTGAGTACG |
| *Mcp1* | CTTCTGGGCCTGCTGTTCA | CCAGCCTACTCATTGGGATCA |
| *Mpo* | TCCCACTCAGCAAGGTCTT | TAAGAGCAGGCAAATCCAG |
| *Nox1* | GGATCCATGGCCTGGGTGGGAT | GGATGCCTGCAACTCCCCTTA |
| *Nox4* | TCCAAGCTCATTTCCCACAG | CGGAGTTCCATTACATCAGAGG |
| *Npc1* | GGGGCATCAGTTACAATGCT | AAACACCGCACTTCCCATAG |
| *Nqo1* | TATCCTTCCGAGTCATCTCTAGCA | TCTGCAGCTTCCAGCTTCTTG |
| *Nrf1* | AGCACGGAGTGACCCAAAC | TGTACGTGGCTACATGGACCT |
| *Pdgf-B* | GCCTGTGACTAGAAGTCCTG | GTCATGGGTGTGCTTAAACT |
| *rCc1* | CCCGGTCAGTTTCAGGATAA | GAAGAGGCTGAAGTTGGTCG |
| *Srebp1c* | GGAGCCATGGATTGCACATT | GCTTCCAGAGAGGAGGCCA |
| *Smad7* | GTTGCTGTGAATCTTACGGG | ATCTGGACAGCCTGCA |
| *Tgfβ* | GTGGAAATCAACGGGATCAG | ACTTCCAACCCAGGTCCTTC |
| *Tnfα* | CCACCACGCTCTTCTGTCTAC | AGGGTCTGGGCCATAGAACT |
| *18S* | TTCGAACGTCTGCCCTATCAA | ATGGTAGGCACGGCGACTA |
| *36B4* | GCAGACAACGTGGGCTCCAAGCAGAT | GGTCCTCCTTGGTGAACACGAAGCCC |

**Table S3: mRNA Analysis of Hepatic Genes in Mice Kept on a Regular Diet**

|  | $Ccl^{+/+}$ | L-CC1 | $Ccl^{-/-}$ | $Ccl^{-/-xliver+}$ |
|---|---|---|---|---|
| **Lipid metabolism** | | | | |
| Srebp1c | 0.8 ± 0.2 | 0.7 ± 0.2 | 2.6 ± 0.4[ab] | 0.5 ± 0.1[c] |
| Fasn | 1.9 ± 0.4 | 1.9 ± 0.3 | 4.0 ± 0.4[ab] | 2.5 ± 0.2[c] |
| Cd36 | 0.6 ± 0.0 | 0.6 ± 0.1 | 1.9 ± 0.1[ab] | 0.8 ± 0.1[c] |
| Fgf21 | 1.2 ± 0.1 | 1.3 ± 0.1 | 0.6 ± 0.0[ab] | 1.2 ± 0.1[c] |
| Cyp2E1 | 0.4 ± 0.3 | 0.4 ± 0.1 | 0.3 ± 0.1 | 0.5 ± 0.2 |
| **Inflammation** | | | | |
| F4/80 | 0.3 ± 0.1 | 0.2 ± 0.1 | 1.4 ± 0.1[ab] | 0.3 ± 0.1[c] |
| Cd68 | 2.3 ± 0.2 | 2.5 ± 0.1 | 5.8 ± 0.2[ab] | 2.3 ± 0.1[c] |
| Mpo | 1.8 ± 0.1 | 1.7 ± 0.1 | 5.0 ± 0.1[ab] | 1.8 ± 0.1[c] |
| Elastase | 1.7 ± 0.1 | 1.6 ± 0.1 | 4.3 ± 0.1[ab] | 1.7 ± 0.1[c] |
| Cd4 | 0.9 ± 0.0 | 1.0 ± 0.1 | 1.7 ± 0.1[ab] | 0.9 ± 0.1[c] |
| Cd8 | 0.5 ± 0.0 | 0.5 ± 0.0 | 1.3 ± 0.1[ab] | 0.5 ± 0.0[c] |
| Foxp3 | 1.0 ± 0.0 | 1.0 ± 0.1 | 0.9 ± 0.1 | 1.0 ± 0.0 |
| Il-10 | 1.6 ± 0.2 | 1.7 ± 0.2 | 1.8 ± 0.1 | 1.8 ± 0.2 |
| Ifnγ | 1.1 ± 0.0 | 1.1 ± 0.1 | 4.8 ± 0.2[ab] | 1.1 ± 0.0[c] |
| Il-4 | 1.9 ± 0.1 | 1.7 ± 0.1 | 1.7 ± 0.1 | 1.9 ± 0.1 |
| Il-13 | 1.5 ± 0.2 | 1.5 ± 0.1 | 1.4 ± 0.1 | 1.3 ± 0.1 |
| Tnfα | 2.4 ± 0.5 | 2.5 ± 0.4 | 5.0 ± 0.5[ab] | 2.5 ± 0.5[c] |
| Il-1β | 0.6 ± 0.1 | 0.6 ± 0.1 | 1.0 ± 0.0[ab] | 0.6 ± 0.1[c] |
| Il-6 | 0.7 ± 0.4 | 0.7 ± 0.4 | 2.6 ± 0.5[ab] | 0.7 ± 0.1[c] |
| Mcp-1/Ccl2 | 0.7 ± 0.1 | 0.7 ± 0.1 | 2.0 ± 0.0[ab] | 0.7 ± 0.1[c] |
| Cd11b | 1.0 ± 0.0 | 1.0 ± 0.0 | 2.5 ± 0.2[ab] | 0.9 ± 0.0[c] |
| Irf8 | 1.0 ± 0.0 | 1.0 ± 0.0 | 0.3 ± 0.0[ab] | 1.0 ± 0.0[c] |
| Gr1 | 1.6 ± 0.0 | 1.6 ± 0.1 | 1.9 ± 0.1 | 1.8 ± 0.1 |
| **Apoptosis** | | | | |
| Chop | 1.0 ± 0.2 | 0.9 ± 0.2 | 1.0 ± 0.2 | 0.8 ± 0.2 |
| Bcl2 | 1.7 ± 0.4 | 1.3 ± 0.4 | 1.8 ± 0.5 | 1.4 ± 0.8 |
| **Hepatocyte Injury** | | | | |
| Hgf | 0.1 ± 0.0 | 0.1 ± 0.2 | 0.4 ± 0.1[ab] | 0.1 ± 0.1[c] |
| Nqo1 | 0.1 ± 0.1 | 0.2 ± 0.1 | 0.6 ± 0.1[ab] | 0.2 ± 0.1[c] |
| Nrf1 | 0.7 ± 0.1 | 0.5 ± 0.1 | 1.6 ± 0.1[ab] | 0.5 ± 0.0[c] |
| **Oxidative Stress** | | | | |
| Nox1 | 0.8 ± 0.0 | 0.8 ± 0.1 | 2.3 ± 0.1[ab] | 0.8 ± 0.1[c] |
| Nox4 | 0.2 ± 0.1 | 0.3 ± 0.0 | 0.8 ± 0.1[ab] | 0.4 ± 0.1[c] |
| Npc1 | 1.0 ± 0.0 | 0.9 ± 0.0 | 1.2 ± 0.1 | 1.2 ± 0.1 |
| Hif1α | 1.5 ± 0.1 | 1.7 ± 0.1 | 4.2 ± 0.1[ab] | 1.4 ± 0.2[c] |
| **Fibrosis** | | | | |
| Smad7 | 1.7 ± 0.4 | 1.6 ± 0.2 | 0.6 ± 0.1[ab] | 1.5 ± 0.1[c] |
| α-Sma | 0.3 ± 0.1 | 0.2 ± 0.1 | 1.2 ± 0.1[ab] | 0.2 ± 0.1[c] |

Livers were extracted from overnight-fasted 6-month-old male mice kept on a regular diet (n≥5 mice/genotype). mRNA content was analyzed by qRT-PCR (normalized to 18S). Values are expressed as mean ± SEM. $^a P<0.05$ *vs Ccl*$^{+/+}$, $^b P<0.05$ *vs* L-CC1, $^c P<0.05$ *vs Ccl*$^{-/-}$.

Table S4: mRNA Analysis of Hepatic Genes in Mice Fed a High-Fat Diet for

3 Months

| | $Ccl^{+/+}$ | L-CC1 | $Ccl^{-/-}$ | $Ccl^{-/-xliver+}$ |
|---|---|---|---|---|
| **Lipid metabolism** | | | | |
| *Srebp1c* | 0.4 ± 0.3 | 0.4 ± 0.1 | 2.2 ± 0.6 [a,b] | 0.3 ± 0.3 [c] |
| *Fasn* | 0.9 ± 0.1 | 0.9 ± 0.2 | 3.9 ± 0.4 [a,b] | 0.7 ± 0.2 [c] |
| *Fgf21* | 2.0 ± 0.3 | 1.9 ± 0.1 | 0.9 ± 0.0 [a,b] | 2.0 ± 0.1 [c] |
| *Cd36* | 0.7 ± 0.1 | 0.9 ± 0.1 | 1.4 ± 0.1 [a,b] | 0.8 ± 0.1 [c] |
| *Cyp2E1* | 1.0 ± 0.2 | 1.2 ± 0.2 | 2.1 ± 0.2 [a,b] | 1.0 ± 0.1 [c] |
| **Inflammation** | | | | |
| *F4/80* | 2.0 ± 0.3 | 0.9 ± 0.4 | 3.9 ± 0.9 [a,b] | 1.9 ± 0.2 [c] |
| *Cd68* | 2.2 ± 0.4 | 2.2 ± 0.1 | 5.6 ± 0.1 [a,b] | 2.6 ± 0.2 [c] |
| *Mpo* | 1.6 ± 0.2 | 1.5 ± 0.2 | 4.4 ± 0.2 [a,b] | 1.6 ± 0.0 [c] |
| *Elastase* | 1.2 ± 0.1 | 1.6 ± 0.2 | 4.1 ± 0.3 [a,b] | 1.6 ± 0.1 [c] |
| *Cd4* | 0.4 ± 0.0 | 0.5 ± 0.0 | 0.9 ± 0.0 [a,b] | 0.4 ± 0.0 [c] |
| *Cd8* | 0.5 ± 0.0 | 0.5 ± 0.0 | 0.9 ± 0.0 [a,b] | 0.5 ± 0.0 [c] |
| *Foxp3* | 0.9 ± 0.0 | 0.8 ± 0.1 | 0.9 ± 0.1 | 0.8 ± 0.1 |
| *Il-10* | 1.5 ± 0.2 | 1.3 ± 0.1 | 1.2 ± 0.1 | 1.4 ± 0.2 |
| *Ifnγ* | 1.3 ± 0.1 | 1.4 ± 0.1 | 6.4 ± 0.3 [a,b] | 1.4 ± 0.2 [c] |
| *Il-4* | 1.0 ± 0.0 | 1.0 ± 0.1 | 1.1 ± 0.0 | 1.1 ± 0.0 |
| *Il-13* | 1.0 ± 0.0 | 1.1 ± 0.1 | 1.1 ± 0.1 | 1.1 ± 0.1 |
| *Tnfα* | 1.8 ± 0.3 | 1.9 ± 0.2 | 3.9 ± 0.0 [a,b] | 1.7 ± 0.4 [c] |
| *Il-1β* | 0.4 ± 0.0 | 0.3 ± 0.1 | 0.8 ± 0.0 [a,b] | 0.3 ± 0.1 [c] |
| *Il-6* | 0.1 ± 0.0 | 0.1 ± 0.0 | 0.9 ± 0.3 [a,b] | 0.1 ± 0.0 [c] |
| *Mcp-1/Ccl2* | 0.8 ± 0.1 | 0.7 ± 0.1 | 2.1 ± 0.1 [a,b] | 0.7 ± 0.1 [c] |
| *Cd11b* | 1.0 ± 0.1 | 0.9 ± 0.1 | 3.0 ± 0.2 [a,b] | 0.9 ± 0.0 [c] |
| *Irf8* | 1.1 ± 0.1 | 1.0 ± 0.1 | 0.5 ± 0.1 [a,b] | 1.0 ± 0.1 [c] |
| *Gr1* | 1.2 ± 0.1 | 1.5 ± 0.2 | 2.7 ± 0.2 [a,b] | 1.6 ± 0.2 [c] |
| **Apoptosis** | | | | |
| *Chop* | 0.3 ± 0.1 | 0.3 ± 0.1 | 0.9 ± 0.0 [a,b] | 0.4 ± 0.1 [c] |
| *Bcl2* | 1.5 ± 0.3 | 1.4 ± 0.2 | 0.3 ± 0.1 [a,b] | 1.7 ± 0.4 [c] |
| **Hepatocyte Injury** | | | | |
| *Hgf* | 1.2 ± 0.2 | 1.8 ± 0.1 | 3.0 ± 0.2 [a,b] | 1.6 ± 0.3 [c] |
| *Nqo1* | 1.2 ± 0.1 | 1.6 ± 0.2 | 3.8 ± 0.5 [a,b] | 2.0 ± 0.4 [c] |
| *Nrf1* | 0.9 ± 0.1 | 1.2 ± 0.2 | 2.1 ± 0.1 [a,b] | 1.1 ± 0.3 [c] |
| **Oxidative Stress** | | | | |
| *Nox1* | 0.8 ± 0.0 | 0.7 ± 0.1 | 2.5 ± 0.1 [a,b] | 0.8 ± 0.1 [c] |
| *Nox4* | 0.9 ± 0.0 | 0.9 ± 0.1 | 1.2 ± 0.2 [a,b] | 0.7 ± 0.0 [c] |
| *Npc1* | 1.3 ± 0.1 | 1.4 ± 0.2 | 0.6 ± 0.0 [a,b] | 1.6 ± 0.1 [c] |
| *Hif1α* | 1.7 ± 0.2 | 1.3 ± 0.1 | 4.4 ± 0.2 [a,b] | 1.4 ± 0.1 [c] |
| **Fibrosis** | | | | |
| *Smad7* | 1.2 ± 0.2 | 1.0 ± 0.1 | 0.3 ± 0.0 [a,b] | 1.1 ± 0.1 [c] |
| *α-Sma* | 0.1 ± 0.1 | 0.2 ± 0.1 | 0.6 ± 0.1 [a,b] | 0.2 ± 0.1 [c] |

Livers were extracted from overnight-fasted male mice that had been fed a HF diet for 3 months starting at 3 months of age (n≥5 mice/genotype). mRNA content was analyzed by qRT-PCR (normalized to 18S). Values are expressed as mean ± SEM. [a]$P<0.05$ vs $Cc1^{+/+}$, [b]$P<0.05$ vs L-CC1, [c]$P<0.05$ vs $Cc1^{-/-}$.

**Table S5: mRNA Analysis of Genes in White Adipose Tissue**

| | $Ccl^{+/+}$ | L-CC1 | $Ccl^{-/-}$ | $Ccl^{-/-xliver+}$ |
|---|---|---|---|---|
| **a) RD** | | | | |
| *F4/80* | $1.4 \pm 0.2$ | $1.3 \pm 0.2$ | $3.4 \pm 0.2$ [ab] | $1.4 \pm 0.1$ [c] |
| *Tnfα* | $1.1 \pm 0.1$ | $1.6 \pm 0.2$ | $4.4 \pm 0.2$ [ab] | $1.5 \pm 0.1$ [c] |
| *Il-6* | $1.1 \pm 0.1$ | $1.3 \pm 0.1$ | $4.2 \pm 0.2$ [ab] | $1.2 \pm 0.1$ [c] |
| *Il-1β* | $1.1 \pm 0.0$ | $1.2 \pm 0.1$ | $3.5 \pm 0.2$ [ab] | $1.2 \pm 0.1$ [c] |
| *Cd68* | $1.0 \pm 0.0$ | $0.9 \pm 0.0$ | $2.6 \pm 0.2$ [ab] | $1.0 \pm 0.1$ [c] |
| *Cd11b* | $1.0 \pm 0.1$ | $1.1 \pm 0.2$ | $4.1 \pm 0.1$ [ab] | $1.1 \pm 0.1$ [c] |
| *Gr1* | $1.1 \pm 0.0$ | $1.1 \pm 0.1$ | $2.8 \pm 0.0$ [ab] | $1.2 \pm 0.1$ [c] |
| **b) HF** | | | | |
| *F4/80* | $1.2 \pm 0.0$ | $1.1 \pm 0.0$ | $3.1 \pm 0.1$ [ab] | $1.1 \pm 0.0$ [c] |
| *Tnfα* | $1.1 \pm 0.1$ | $1.3 \pm 0.2$ | $4.1 \pm 0.1$ [ab] | $1.1 \pm 0.1$ [c] |
| *Il-6* | $1.2 \pm 0.0$ | $1.4 \pm 0.1$ | $4.3 \pm 0.2$ [ab] | $1.2 \pm 0.1$ [c] |
| *Il-1β* | $0.9 \pm 0.1$ | $1.1 \pm 0.1$ | $3.1 \pm 0.2$ [ab] | $1.0 \pm 0.1$ [c] |
| *Cd68* | $0.9 \pm 0.0$ | $0.9 \pm 0.0$ | $2.6 \pm 0.1$ [ab] | $0.8 \pm 0.1$ [c] |
| *Cd11b* | $2.1 \pm 0.3$ | $1.8 \pm 0.1$ | $3.9 \pm 0.2$ [ab] | $1.5 \pm 0.2$ [c] |
| *Gr1* | $1.2 \pm 0.1$ | $1.5 \pm 0.2$ | $2.7 \pm 0.2$ [ab] | $1.6 \pm 0.2$ [c] |

Male mice (n≥5 mice/genotype) were kept on a regular diet for 6 months or fed a HF diet in their last 3 months before being fasted overnight and their white adipose depot (gonadal plus inguinal) collected to measure mRNA content by qRT-PCR (normalized to 36B4). Values are expressed as mean ± SEM. [a]*P<0.05 vs Ccl$^{+/+}$*, [b]*P<0.05 vs L-CC1*, [c]*P<0.05 vs Ccl$^{-/-}$*.

# A. Western analysis of liver lysates

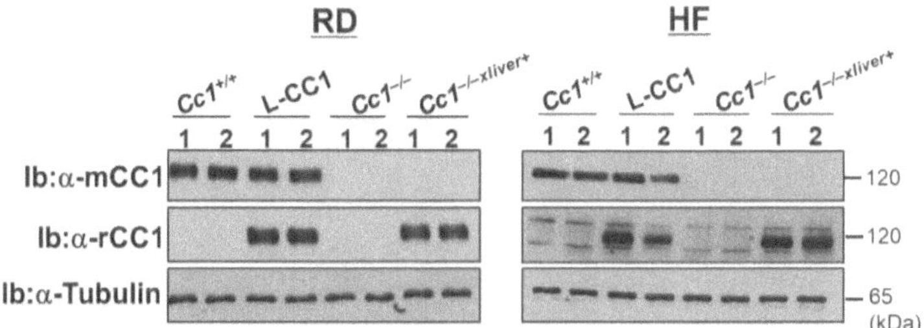


# B. Glucose and insulin tolerance tests

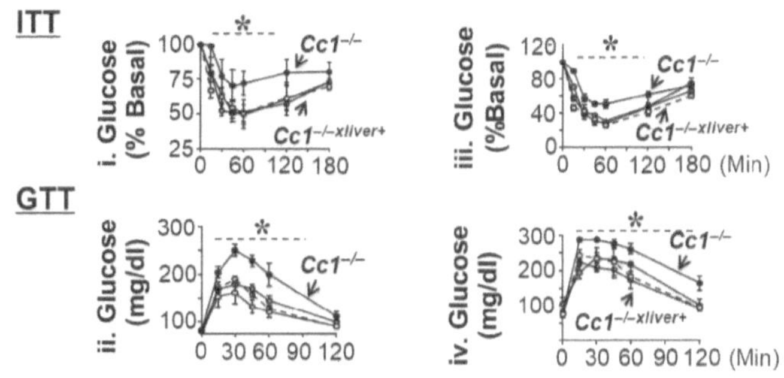

## A. H&E stain

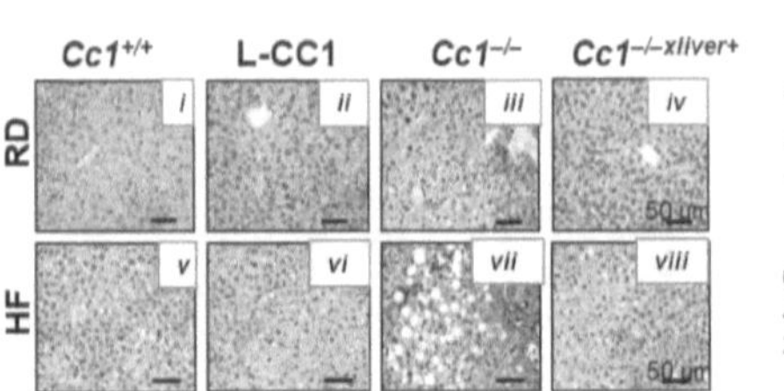


## B. Lipid metabolism

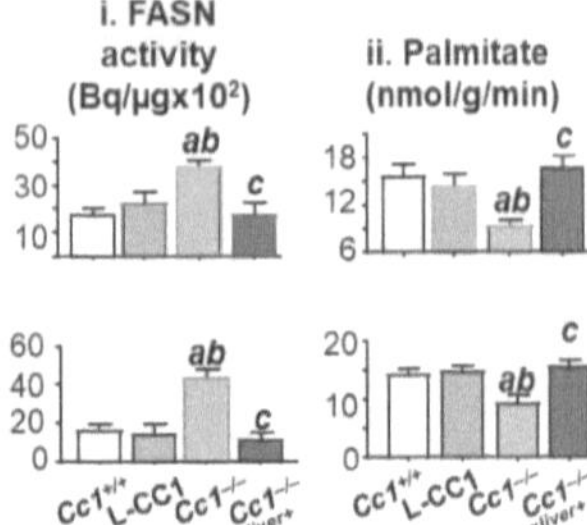


## C. Western blot

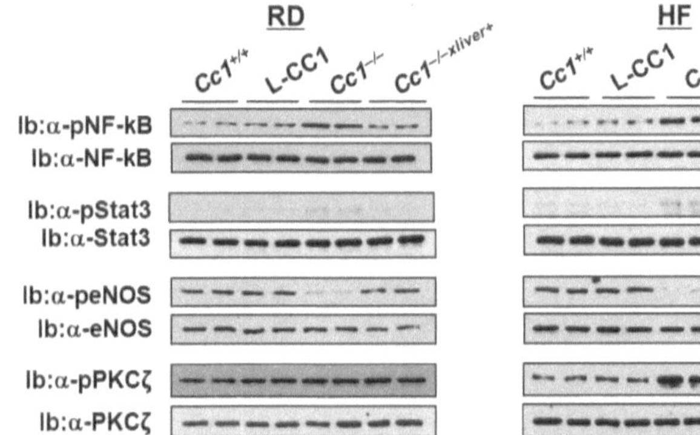


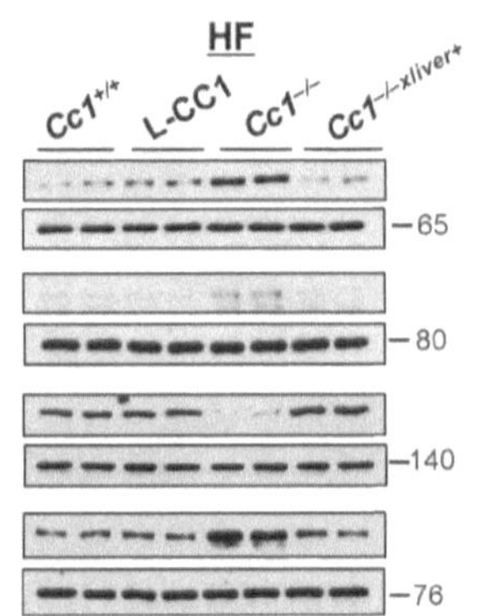


## D. Apoptosis

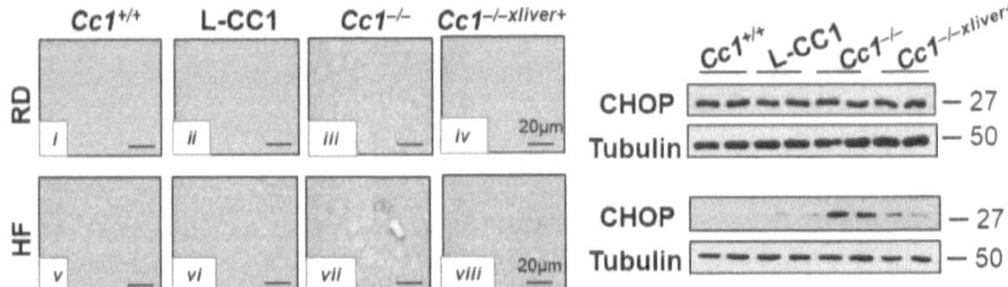

Figure 3

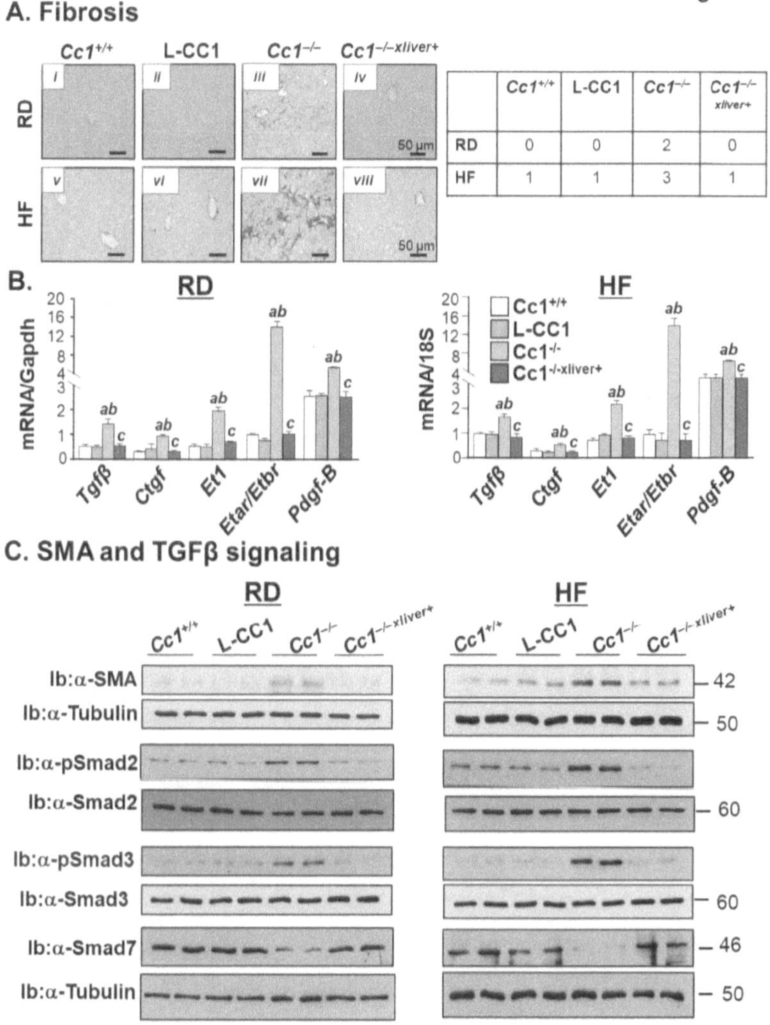


| | Cc1+/+ | L-CC1 | Cc1−/− | Cc1−/− xliver+ |
|---|---|---|---|---|
| RD | 0 | 0 | 2 | 0 |
| HF | 1 | 1 | 3 | 1 |

# Figure S1

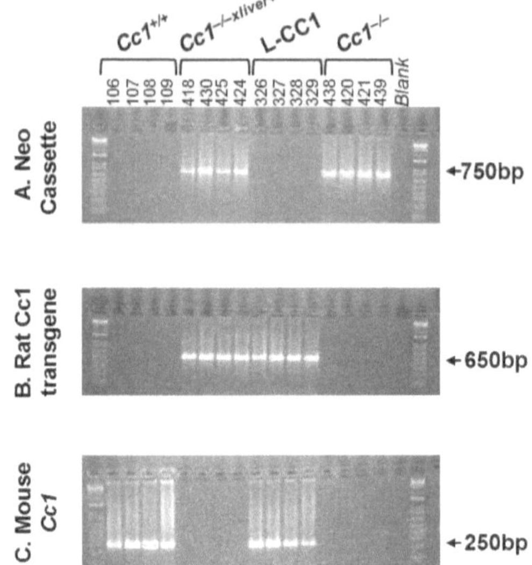



| Gene | ID | Primer sequence (5'-3') |
|---|---|---|
| A. Neo Cassette (Global Cc1 null) | SNeo9 (sense) | GGA TCG GCC ATT GAA GAA GAT |
| | SNeo8 (anti-sense) | CGC CAA GCT CTT CAG CAA TAT |
| B. Rat Ceacam1 transgene (L-CC1) | ALP WT-CC1 TRANSGENIC | GGG CGA ATT GGG TAC ACT TA |
| | R1P WT-CC1 TRANSGENIC | ATA GCA GCG CTG GCA TAC TT |
| C. Mouse Wild-type Ceacam1 | PN8 | CTGCCCCTGGCGCTTGGA |
| | PN5 | TACATGAAATCGCACAGTCGC |

## Chapter 4: Summary, Conclusion and Discussion

Metabolic syndrome is a cluster of medical conditions associated with obesity and sedentary lifestyle. It includes excess fat deposition in the abdominal area, liver, and blood vessels. These conditions increase the risk of cardiovascular disease, non-alcoholic fatty liver disease (NAFLD), and type 2 diabetes. Metabolic syndrome is associated with 68% increased risk of sudden death [157], largely due to cardiovascular failure.

The incidence of NAFLD is on an epidemic rise, affecting more than 17-33% of the general population worldwide [158]. NAFLD is considered as the hepatic manifestation of metabolic syndrome and is basically underlined by insulin resistance. Untreated NAFLD progresses to nonalcoholic steatohepatitis (NASH), the features of which include inflammation, fibrosis, and apoptosis (death) of hepatocytes. NASH, in turn, can progress to cirrhosis and liver adenocarcinoma [159], which constitutes a leading cause of liver transplant globally and in particular in the United States.

Despite its increased incidence, there is no FDA-approved drug targeting this disease, in part because of our limited understanding of how it develops, in particular fibrosis. Weight reduction and insulin sensitizers have been the only therapy for patients with NASH; however, patients regain weight [77] and some gain weight on some insulin sensitizers like PPAR$\gamma$ agonists.

Cardiovascular disease, like atherosclerosis, is the most common cause of death accounting for an estimate of 31.5% of global deaths. Individuals with metabolic syndrome are more susceptible to atherosclerosis. Clinical studies have shown that lowering plasma cholesterol levels does not totally limit the progression of atherosclerosis. This means that cholesterol lowering drugs only treat symptoms without blunting the cause of atherosclerosis. This restrictive practice emerges from our limited understanding of the pathogenesis of the disease, owing in part, to the lack of animal models that replicate faithfully the disease in humans. Future therapeutics against atherosclerosis should directly address the mechanisms driving this fibrotic disease, in particular the pro-inflammatory state [160].

The Najjar laboratory is among the leading laboratories that show that NASH and atherosclerosis are a twin disease, sharing a common etiology [133]. Thus, blunting atherosclerosis requires the development of effective therapeutic modalities against NAFLD/NASH.

Our studies focus on understanding how a protein called Carcinoembryonic antigen-related cell adhesion molecule 1 (CEACAM1) links NAFLD/NASH to atherosclerosis, and how dietary factors, in particular high-calorie intake, reduces CEACAM1 expression and function in the liver to cause these cardiometabolic abnormalities.

CEACAM1 is a transmembrane glycoprotein that is expressed in many tissues including liver, vascular endothelium, and cardiac tissue. It constitutes many important roles in promoting insulin clearance to regulate insulin sensitivity [2] and maintaining vascular homeostasis [48] and proper immune response [1, 86]. Moreover, CEACAM1 protects the liver against the high level of insulin in the portal circulation to prevent excessive fat production under normal physiologic conditions [12].

Studies in genetically modified mice have shown that disturbed function or expression of CEACAM1 leads to insulin resistance and increased fat accumulation in the liver [89]. In addition, mice with total or liver-specific deletion of *Ceacam1* gene manifest insulin resistance, hepatic fibrosis, inflammation and apoptosis [72, 87, 88]. On the other hand, restoring CEACAM1 in the liver rescues the metabolic phenotype of the global null mouse, and redelivering CEACAM1 to the liver prevents insulin resistance and obesity in response to high-fat diet [90]. Moreover, global *Ceacam1* null mice manifest spontaneous cardiac dysfunction together with pre-atherogenic lesions in the aorta [9]. Interestingly, restoring CEACAM1 in the liver reverses these cardiovascular abnormalities in the global null mice [161] even when mice have been fed a high-fat diet. Collectively, this emphasizes the significance of how induction of hepatic CEACAM1 reverses diet-induced insulin resistance, NASH and its cardiovascular correlates.

Because CEACAM1 is also expressed in endothelial cells, studying its role in these cells identified novel means of endothelial CEACAM1 in the pathogenesis of liver fibrosis and atherosclerosis. Studies on mice with conditional loss of endothelial CEACAM1 backcrossed with low-density lipoprotein receptor deficient mice (*ldlr$^{-/-}$ VECad+Ccl$^{fl/fl}$*) showed augmented vascular cell permeability leading to inflammation and the development of fibrotic plaques without aortic lipid deposition. Deleting CEACAM1 from endothelial cells did not alter insulin sensitivity but caused moderate hypercholesterolemia. However, these mutant mice exhibited decreased nitric oxide bioavailability with a reciprocal increase in plasma endothelin 1. Mechanistically, without CEACAM1 in endothelial cells, endothelin-1 levels are elevated, stemming from increased ras-MAPKinase-NF-kB signaling pathways in response to lower sequestration of Shc and increased coupling of Grb2 to insulin and VEGFR2. Activated NF-kB could induce pro-inflammation and with the release of endothelin-1 and PDGF-B, lead to pro-fibrogenesis. Moreover, in the absence of CEACAM1, binding of Shp2 phosphatase to IRS1 (insulin) or VEFGR2 (VEGF) increases to downregulate IRS-1/AKT/eNOS or VEGFR2/AKT/eNOS activity and subsequently, lower nitric oxide production.  Thus, the endothelial cell-specific CEACAM1 knockout can be used to pinpoint how inflammatory-dependent fibrogenesis can develop independently of systemic risk factors (such as hyperinsulinemia and insulin resistance). The development of overt NASH and atherosclerosis (hepatic macrosteatosis and lipid deposition on the aortic wall) in the presence of insulin resistance in mice with liver-specific *Ceacam1* deletion [133] supports the conclusion that insulin resistance is critical in the development of NASH and its link to atherosclerosis.

Of translational relevance, obese patients with NAFLD/NASH display a remarkable decrease in their hepatic CEACAM1 levels and lower insulin clearance has emerged as a major risk factor for metabolic syndrome. Thus, research on CEACAM1 provides in-depth information on how genetics and diet interact during the course of these cardiometabolic abnormalities and how modifying CEACAM1 expression can be used as a therapeutic modality to reverse or prevent the course of these cardiometabolic diseases.

**References**

1.      Heinrich, G., et al., *Loss of Hepatic CEACAM1: A Unifying Mechanism Linking Insulin Resistance to Obesity and Non-Alcoholic Fatty Liver Disease.* Front Endocrinol (Lausanne), 2017. 8: p. 8.

2.      Najjar, S.M., *Regulation of insulin action by CEACAM1.* Trends Endocrinol Metab, 2002. 13(6): p. 240-5.

3.      Ghavampour, S., et al., *Endothelial barrier function is differentially regulated by CEACAM1-mediated signaling.* FASEB J, 2018. 32(10): p. 5612-5625.

4.      Obrink, B., *CEA adhesion molecules: multifunctional proteins with signal-regulatory properties.* Curr Opin Cell Biol, 1997. 9(5): p. 616-26.

5.      Liu, J., et al., *Loss of Ceacam1 promotes prostate cancer progression in Pten haploinsufficient male mice.* Metabolism, 2020. 107: p. 154215.

6.      Gray-Owen, S.D. and R.S. Blumberg, *CEACAM1: contact-dependent control of immunity.* Nat Rev Immunol, 2006. 6(6): p. 433-46.

7.      Bergman, R.N., et al., *Hypothesis: Role of Reduced Hepatic Insulin Clearance in the Pathogenesis of Type 2 Diabetes.* Diabetes, 2019. 68(9): p. 1709-1716.

8.      Gu, A., et al., *Generation of Human CEACAM1 Transgenic Mice and Binding of Neisseria Opa Protein to Their Neutrophils.* Plos One, 2010. 5(4).

9.      Najjar, S.M., et al., *Ceacam1 deletion causes vascular alterations in large vessels.* Am J Physiol Endocrinol Metab, 2013. 305(4): p. E519-29.

10.     Rosenfeld, L., *Insulin: Discovery and controversy.* Clinical Chemistry, 2002. 48(12): p. 2270-2288.

11.     Fu, Z., E.R. Gilbert, and D. Liu, *Regulation of insulin synthesis and secretion and pancreatic Beta-cell dysfunction in diabetes.* Curr Diabetes Rev, 2013. 9(1): p. 25-53.

12.     Najjar, S.M. and G. Perdomo, *Hepatic Insulin Clearance: Mechanism and Physiology.* Physiology, 2019. 34(3): p. 198-215.

13.     Kahn, C.R., *The Molecular Mechanism of Insulin Action.* Annual Review of Medicine, 1985. 36: p. 429-451.

14.     Rajwani, A., R.M. Cubbon, and S.B. Wheatcroft, *Cell-specific insulin resistance: implications for atherosclerosis.* Diabetes Metab Res Rev, 2012. 28(8): p. 627-34.

15.     Rask-Madsen, C., et al., *Loss of insulin signaling in vascular endothelial cells accelerates atherosclerosis in apolipoprotein E null mice.* Cell Metab, 2010. 11(5): p. 379-89.

16.     Tsuchiya, K., et al., *FoxOs integrate pleiotropic actions of insulin in vascular endothelium to protect mice from atherosclerosis.* Cell Metab, 2012. 15(3): p. 372-81.

17.     Tanaka, J., et al., *Foxo1 links hyperglycemia to LDL oxidation and endothelial nitric oxide synthase dysfunction in vascular endothelial cells.* Diabetes, 2009. 58(10): p. 2344-54.

18.     Kiriakidis, S., et al., *VEGF expression in human macrophages is NF-kappaB-dependent: studies using adenoviruses expressing the endogenous NF-kappaB inhibitor IkappaBalpha and a kinase-defective form of the IkappaB kinase 2.* J Cell Sci, 2003. 116(Pt 4): p. 665-74.

19.     Wagener, C. and S. Ergun, *Angiogenic properties of the carcinoembryonic antigen-related cell adhesion molecule 1.* Exp Cell Res, 2000. 261(1): p. 19-24.

20.     E, G., et al., *Endogenous vascular endothelial growth factor-A (VEGF-A) maintains endothelial cell homeostasis by regulating VEGF receptor-2 transcription.* J Biol Chem, 2012. 287(5): p. 3029-41.

21.     Tabruyn, S.P. and A.W. Griffioen, *NF-kappa B: a new player in angiostatic therapy.* Angiogenesis, 2008. 11(1): p. 101-6.

22.     Gimbrone, M.A., Jr. and G. Garcia-Cardena, *Endothelial Cell Dysfunction and the Pathobiology of Atherosclerosis.* Circ Res, 2016. 118(4): p. 620-36.

23.     Di Pino, A. and R.A. DeFronzo, *Insulin Resistance and Atherosclerosis: Implications for Insulin-Sensitizing Agents.* Endocr Rev, 2019. 40(6): p. 1447-1467.

24.     Tousoulis, D., et al., *The role of nitric oxide on endothelial function.* Curr Vasc Pharmacol, 2012. 10(1): p. 4-18.

25.     Davignon, J. and P. Ganz, *Role of endothelial dysfunction in atherosclerosis.* Circulation, 2004. 109(23 Suppl 1): p. III27-32.

26.     Fan, J.L., et al., *Role of endothelin-1 in atherosclerosis.* Atherosclerosis V: The Fifth Saratoga Conference, 2000. 902: p. 84-94.

27.     Kuprash, D.V. and S.A. Nedospasov, *Molecular and Cellular Mechanisms of Inflammation.* Biochemistry (Mosc), 2016. 81(11): p. 1237-1239.

28.     Weiskirchen, R., S. Weiskirchen, and F. Tacke, *Organ and tissue fibrosis: Molecular signals, cellular mechanisms and translational implications.* Mol Aspects Med, 2019. 65: p. 2-15.

29.     Medzhitov, R., *Origin and physiological roles of inflammation.* Nature, 2008. 454(7203): p. 428-35.

30.     Mierke, C.T., *The fundamental role of mechanical properties in the progression of cancer disease and inflammation.* Rep Prog Phys, 2014. 77(7): p. 076602.

31.     Assar, M.E., J. Angulo, and L. Rodriguez-Manas, *Diabetes and ageing-induced vascular inflammation.* J Physiol, 2016. 594(8): p. 2125-46.

32.     Zhu, Y., et al., *Research Progress on the Relationship between Atherosclerosis and Inflammation.* Biomolecules, 2018. 8(3).

33.     Qamar, A. and D.J. Rader, *Effect of interleukin 1beta inhibition in cardiovascular disease.* Curr Opin Lipidol, 2012. 23(6): p. 548-53.

34.     Alaarg, A., et al., *A systematic comparison of clinically viable nanomedicines targeting HMG-CoA reductase in inflammatory atherosclerosis.* J Control Release, 2017. 262: p. 47-57.

35.     Rasic, S., et al., *Influence of Malondialdehyde and Matrix Metalloproteinase-9 on Progression of Carotid Atherosclerosis in Chronic Renal Disease with Cardiometabolic Syndrome.* Mediators Inflamm, 2015. 2015: p. 614357.

36.     Zapolska-Downar, D., et al., *Simvastatin modulates TNFalpha-induced adhesion molecules expression in human endothelial cells.* Life Sci, 2004. 75(11): p. 1287-302.

37.     Wegermann, K., A.M. Diehl, and C.A. Moylan, *Disease pathways and molecular mechanisms of nonalcoholic steatohepatitis.* Clin Liver Dis (Hoboken), 2018. 11(4): p. 87-91.

38.     Ghadieh, H.E., et al., *Loss of Hepatic Carcinoembryonic Antigen-Related Cell Adhesion Molecule 1 Links Nonalcoholic Steatohepatitis to Atherosclerosis.* Hepatol Commun, 2020. 4(11): p. 1591-1609.

39.     Bessone, F., M.V. Razori, and M.G. Roma, *Molecular pathways of nonalcoholic fatty liver disease development and progression.* Cell Mol Life Sci, 2019. 76(1): p. 99-128.

40.     Mack, M., *Inflammation and fibrosis.* Matrix Biol, 2018. 68-69: p. 106-121.

41.     Benjamin, E.J., et al., *Heart Disease and Stroke Statistics-2017 Update: A Report From the American Heart Association.* Circulation, 2017. 135(10): p. e146-e603.

42.     Ross, R., *The pathogenesis of atherosclerosis: a perspective for the 1990s.* Nature, 1993. 362(6423): p. 801-9.

43.     Galkina, E. and K. Ley, *Immune and inflammatory mechanisms of atherosclerosis (*).* Annu Rev Immunol, 2009. 27: p. 165-97.

44.     Frank, P.G. and M.P. Lisanti, *ICAM-1: role in inflammation and in the regulation of vascular permeability.* Am J Physiol Heart Circ Physiol, 2008. 295(3): p. H926-H927.

45.     Jeong, J., et al., *Soluble RAGE attenuates AngII-induced endothelial hyperpermeability by disrupting HMGB1-mediated crosstalk between AT1R and RAGE.* Exp Mol Med, 2019. 51(9): p. 113.

46.	Varghese, J.F., R. Patel, and U.C.S. Yadav, *Novel insights in the metabolic syndrome-induced oxidative stress and inflammation-mediated atherosclerosis.* Curr Cardiol Rev, 2017.

47.	Reglero-Real, N., et al., *Endothelial Cell Junctional Adhesion Molecules: Role and Regulation of Expression in Inflammation.* Arterioscler Thromb Vasc Biol, 2016. 36(10): p. 2048-2057.

48.	Rueckschloss, U., S. Kuerten, and S. Ergun, *The role of CEA-related cell adhesion molecule-1 (CEACAM1) in vascular homeostasis.* Histochem Cell Biol, 2016. 146(6): p. 657-671.

49.	Gerstel, D., et al., *CEACAM1 creates a pro-angiogenic tumor microenvironment that supports tumor vessel maturation.* Oncogene, 2011. 30(41): p. 4275-4288.

50.	Usman, A., et al., *From Lipid Retention to Immune-Mediate Inflammation and Associated Angiogenesis in the Pathogenesis of Atherosclerosis.* J Atheroscler Thromb, 2015. 22(8): p. 739-49.

51.	Schulze, P.C., K. Drosatos, and I.J. Goldberg, *Lipid Use and Misuse by the Heart.* Circulation Research, 2016. 118(11): p. 1736-1751.

52.	Linton, M.R.F., et al., *The Role of Lipids and Lipoproteins in Atherosclerosis*, in *Endotext*, K.R. Feingold, et al., Editors. 2000: South Dartmouth (MA).

53.	Sakurai, T., et al., *Measurement of lipoprotein particle sizes using dynamic light scattering.* Ann Clin Biochem, 2010. 47(Pt 5): p. 476-81.

54.    Chen, Q., et al., *Association of anti-oxidized LDL and candidate genes with severity of coronary stenosis in the Women's Ischemia Syndrome Evaluation study.* J Lipid Res, 2011. 52(4): p. 801-7.

55.    Tabas, I., K.J. Williams, and J. Boren, *Subendothelial lipoprotein retention as the initiating process in atherosclerosis - Update and therapeutic implications.* Circulation, 2007. 116(16): p. 1832-1844.

56.    Neeland, I.J., P. Poirier, and J.P. Despres, *Cardiovascular and Metabolic Heterogeneity of Obesity: Clinical Challenges and Implications for Management.* Circulation, 2018. 137(13): p. 1391-1406.

57.    Petersen, K.F. and G.I. Shulman, *Etiology of insulin resistance.* American Journal of Medicine, 2006. 119(5): p. 10s-16s.

58.    Wakil, S.J. and L.A. Abu-Elheiga, *Fatty acid metabolism: target for metabolic syndrome.* Journal of Lipid Research, 2009. 50: p. S138-S143.

59.    Leone, T.C., C.J. Weinheimer, and D.P. Kelly, *A critical role for the peroxisome proliferator-activated receptor alpha (PPARalpha) in the cellular fasting response: the PPARalpha-null mouse as a model of fatty acid oxidation disorders.* Proc Natl Acad Sci U S A, 1999. 96(13): p. 7473-8.

60.    Ramakrishnan, S.K., et al., *PPARalpha (Peroxisome Proliferator-activated Receptor alpha) Activation Reduces Hepatic CEACAM1 Protein Expression to Regulate Fatty Acid Oxidation during Fasting-refeeding Transition.* J Biol Chem, 2016. 291(15): p. 8121-9.

61.     Evans, R.M., G.D. Barish, and Y.X. Wang, *PPARs and the complex journey to obesity.* Nat Med, 2004. 10(4): p. 355-61.

62.     Kersten, S., et al., *Peroxisome proliferator-activated receptor alpha mediates the adaptive response to fasting.* J Clin Invest, 1999. 103(11): p. 1489-98.

63.     Najjar, S.M., et al., *Insulin acutely decreases hepatic fatty acid synthase activity.* Cell Metab, 2005. 2(1): p. 43-53.

64.     Najjar, S.M. and G. Perdomo, *Hepatic Insulin Clearance: Mechanism and Physiology.* Physiology (Bethesda), 2019. 34(3): p. 198-215.

65.     Najjar, S.M., *The Lipogenic Effect of Insulin Revisited*, in *Hepatic De Novo Lipogenesis and Regulation of Metabolism*, J.M. Ntambi, Editor. 2016, Springer International Publishing: Cham. p. 285-295.

66.     Jia, G., V.G. DeMarco, and J.R. Sowers, *Insulin resistance and hyperinsulinaemia in diabetic cardiomyopathy.* Nat Rev Endocrinol, 2016. 12(3): p. 144-53.

67.     Chen, W., E. Balland, and M.A. Cowley, *Hypothalamic Insulin Resistance in Obesity: Effects on Glucose Homeostasis.* Neuroendocrinology, 2017. 104(4): p. 364-381.

68.     Hong, F., et al., *PPARs as Nuclear Receptors for Nutrient and Energy Metabolism.* Molecules, 2019. 24(14).

69.     Tokarz, V.L., P.E. MacDonald, and A. Klip, *The cell biology of systemic insulin function.* J Cell Biol, 2018. 217(7): p. 2273-2289.

70. Thomas, D.D., et al., *Hyperinsulinemia: An Early Indicator of Metabolic Dysfunction.* J Endocr Soc, 2019. 3(9): p. 1727-1747.

71. Poy, M.N., et al., *CEACAM1 regulates insulin clearance in liver.* Nat Genet, 2002. 30(3): p. 270-6.

72. Ghadieh, H.E., et al., *Hyperinsulinemia drives hepatic insulin resistance in male mice with liver-specific Ceacam1 deletion independently of lipolysis.* Metabolism, 2019. 93: p. 33-43.

73. Watt, M.J., et al., *The Liver as an Endocrine Organ-Linking NAFLD and Insulin Resistance.* Endocr Rev, 2019. 40(5): p. 1367-1393.

74. Gastaldelli, A. and K. Cusi, *From NASH to diabetes and from diabetes to NASH: Mechanisms and treatment options.* JHEP Rep, 2019. 1(4): p. 312-328.

75. Zimmet, P., et al., *Etiology of the Metabolic Syndrome: Potential role of insulin resistance, leptin resistance, and other players.* The Metabolic Syndrome X, 1999. 892: p. 25-44.

76. Perry, R.J., et al., *The role of hepatic lipids in hepatic insulin resistance and type 2 diabetes.* Nature, 2014. 510(7503): p. 84-91.

77. Najjar, S.M. and L. Russo, *CEACAM1 loss links inflammation to insulin resistance in obesity and non-alcoholic steatohepatitis (NASH).* Semin Immunopathol, 2014. 36(1): p. 55-71.

78. Jennings, J., C. Faselis, and M.D. Yao, *NAFLD-NASH: An Under-Recognized Epidemic.* Curr Vasc Pharmacol, 2018. 16(3): p. 209-213.

79.     Younossi, Z.M., et al., *Global Epidemiology of Nonalcoholic Fatty Liver Disease-Meta-Analytic Assessment of Prevalence, Incidence, and Outcomes.* Hepatology, 2016. 64(1): p. 73-84.

80.     Estes, C., et al., *Modeling the epidemic of nonalcoholic fatty liver disease demonstrates an exponential increase in burden of disease.* Hepatology, 2018. 67(1): p. 123-133.

81.     Di Conza, G. and P.C. Ho, *ER Stress Responses: An Emerging Modulator for Innate Immunity.* Cells, 2020. 9(3).

82.     Jung, K.Y., et al., *Nonalcoholic steatohepatitis associated with metabolic syndrome: relationship to insulin resistance and liver histology.* J Clin Gastroenterol, 2014. 48(10): p. 883-8.

83.     Czaja, A.J., *Hepatic inflammation and progressive liver fibrosis in chronic liver disease.* World J Gastroenterol, 2014. 20(10): p. 2515-32.

84.     Rozpedek, W., et al., *The Role of the PERK/eIF2alpha/ATF4/CHOP Signaling Pathway in Tumor Progression During Endoplasmic Reticulum Stress.* Curr Mol Med, 2016. 16(6): p. 533-44.

85.     Xu, M., et al., *Key role of liver sinusoidal endothelial cells in liver fibrosis.* Biosci Trends, 2017. 11(2): p. 163-168.

86.     Horst, A.K., et al., *CEACAM1 in Liver Injury, Metabolic and Immune Regulation.* Int J Mol Sci, 2018. 19(10).

87.    DeAngelis, A.M., et al., *Carcinoembryonic antigen-related cell adhesion molecule 1 - A link between insulin and lipid metabolism.* Diabetes, 2008. 57(9): p. 2296-2303.

88.    Ghosh, S., et al., *Mice with null mutation of Ceacam 1 develop nonalcoholic steatohepatitis.* Hepat Med, 2010. 2010(2): p. 69-78.

89.    Lee, S.J., et al., *Development of nonalcoholic steatohepatitis in insulin-resistant liver-specific S503A carcinoembryonic antigen-related cell adhesion molecule 1 mutant mice.* Gastroenterology, 2008. 135(6): p. 2084-95.

90.    Russo, L., et al., *Liver-specific reconstitution of CEACAM1 reverses the metabolic abnormalities caused by its global deletion in male mice.* Diabetologia, 2017. 60(12): p. 2463-2474.

91.    Rask-Madsen, C., et al., *Hyperinsulinemia does not change atherosclerosis development in apolipoprotein E null mice.* Arterioscler Thromb Vasc Biol, 2012. 32(5): p. 1124-31.

92.    Khalil, M.F., W.D. Wagner, and I.J. Goldberg, *Molecular interactions leading to lipoprotein retention and the initiation of atherosclerosis.* Arterioscler Thromb Vasc Biol, 2004. 24(12): p. 2211-8.

93.    Vita, J.A., et al., *Coronary vasomotor response to acetylcholine relates to risk factors for coronary artery disease.* Circulation, 1990. 81(2): p. 491-7.

94.    Russo, L., et al., *Role for hepatic CEACAM1 in regulating fatty acid metabolism along the adipocyte-hepatocyte axis.* J Lipid Res, 2016. 57(12): p. 2163-2175.

95.     Li, Y., et al., *A novel role for CRTC2 in hepatic cholesterol synthesis through SREBP-2.* Hepatology, 2017. 66(2): p. 481-497.

96.     Marchio, P., et al., *Targeting Early Atherosclerosis: A Focus on Oxidative Stress and Inflammation.* Oxid Med Cell Longev, 2019. 2019: p. 8563845.

97.     Li, B., et al., *Inflammation: A Novel Therapeutic Target/Direction in Atherosclerosis.* Curr Pharm Des, 2017. 23(8): p. 1216-1227.

98.     Chen, Q., et al., *Targeted inhibition of STAT3 as a potential treatment strategy for atherosclerosis.* Theranostics, 2019. 9(22): p. 6424-6442.

99.     Ueda, Y., et al., *Reduction of 8-iso-prostaglandin F2alpha in the first week after Roux-en-Y gastric bypass surgery.* Obesity (Silver Spring), 2011. 19(8): p. 1663-8.

100.    Meng, L.B., et al., *Common Injuries and Repair Mechanisms in the Endothelial Lining.* Chin Med J (Engl), 2018. 131(19): p. 2338-2345.

101.    Satitthummanid, S., et al., *Depleted nitric oxide and prostaglandin E2 levels are correlated with endothelial dysfunction in beta-thalassemia/HbE patients.* Int J Hematol, 2017. 106(3): p. 366-374.

102.    Chistiakov, D.A., A.N. Orekhov, and Y.V. Bobryshev, *Endothelial Barrier and Its Abnormalities in Cardiovascular Disease.* Front Physiol, 2015. 6: p. 365.

103.    Wang, H.H., et al., *Cholesterol and Lipoprotein Metabolism and Atherosclerosis: Recent Advances In reverse Cholesterol Transport.* Ann Hepatol, 2017. 16(0): p. 21-36.

104.    Goldberg, I.J., *Why does diabetes increase atherosclerosis? I don't know!* Journal of Clinical Investigation, 2004. 114(5): p. 613-615.

105.    Hartvigsen, K., et al., *A diet-induced hypercholesterolemic murine model to study atherogenesis without obesity and metabolic syndrome.* Arteriosclerosis Thrombosis and Vascular Biology, 2007. 27(4): p. 878-885.

106.    Wu, L., et al., *Addition of dietary fat to cholesterol in the diets of LDL receptor knockout mice: effects on plasma insulin, lipoproteins, and atherosclerosis.* J Lipid Res, 2006. 47(10): p. 2215-22.

107.    Camare, C., et al., *Angiogenesis in the atherosclerotic plaque.* Redox Biol, 2017. 12: p. 18-34.

108.    Badimon, L. and G. Vilahur, *Thrombosis formation on atherosclerotic lesions and plaque rupture.* J Intern Med, 2014. 276(6): p. 618-32.

109.    Virmani, R., et al., *Lessons from sudden coronary death: a comprehensive morphological classification scheme for atherosclerotic lesions.* Arterioscler Thromb Vasc Biol, 2000. 20(5): p. 1262-75.

110.    Goldberg, I.J., et al., *Decreased lipoprotein clearance is responsible for increased cholesterol in LDL receptor knockout mice with streptozotocin-induced diabetes.* Diabetes, 2008. 57(6): p. 1674-1682.

111.    Horton, J.D., J.C. Cohen, and H.H. Hobbs, *PCSK9: a convertase that coordinates LDL catabolism.* Journal of Lipid Research, 2009. 50: p. S172-S177.

112.  Canuel, M., et al., *Proprotein Convertase Subtilisin/Kexin Type 9 (PCSK9) Can Mediate Degradation of the Low Density Lipoprotein Receptor-Related Protein 1 (LRP-1).* Plos One, 2013. 8(5).

113.  Buzzetti, E., M. Pinzani, and E.A. Tsochatzis, *The multiple-hit pathogenesis of non-alcoholic fatty liver disease (NAFLD).* Metabolism, 2016. 65(8): p. 1038-48.

114.  Younossi, Z.M., *Non-alcoholic fatty liver disease - A global public health perspective.* J. Hepatol., 2019. 70(3): p. 531-544.

115.  Tilg, H. and A.R. Moschen, *Evolution of inflammation in nonalcoholic fatty liver disease: the multiple parallel hits hypothesis.* Hepatology, 2010. 52(5): p. 1836-46.

116.  Gan, L.T., et al., *Hepatocyte free cholesterol lipotoxicity results from JNK1-mediated mitochondrial injury and is HMGB1 and TLR4-dependent.* J. Hepatol., 2014. 61(6): p. 1376-84.

117.  Fuchs, M. and A.J. Sanyal, *Lipotoxicity in NASH.* J. Hepatol., 2012. 56(1): p. 291-3.

118.  Dallio, M., et al., *Immunity as Cornerstone of Non-Alcoholic Fatty Liver Disease: The Contribution of Oxidative Stress in the Disease Progression.* Int. J. Mol. Sci., 2021. 22(1).

119.  Masarone, M., et al., *Role of Oxidative Stress in Pathophysiology of Nonalcoholic Fatty Liver Disease.* Oxid Med Cell Longev, 2018. 2018: p. 9547613.

120.  Thomas, D.D., et al., *Hyperinsulinemia: An Early Indicator of Metabolic Dysfunction.* J. Endocr. Soc., 2019. 3(9): p. 1727-1747.

121.	Gastaldelli, A. and K. Cusi, *From NASH to diabetes and from diabetes to NASH: Mechanisms and treatment options.* JHEP Rep., 2019. 1(4): p. 312-328.

122.	Stefan, N., H.U. Haring, and K. Cusi, *Non-alcoholic fatty liver disease: causes, diagnosis, cardiometabolic consequences, and treatment strategies.* Lancet Diabetes Endocrinol., 2019. 7(4): p. 313-324.

123.	Bril, F., et al., *Relationship Between Disease Severity, Hyperinsulinemia, and Impaired Insulin Clearance in Patients With Nonalcoholic Steatohepatitis.* Hepatology, 2014. 59(6): p. 2178-2187.

124.	Heinrich, G., et al., *Reduced hepatic carcinoembryonic antigen-related cell adhesion molecule 1 level in obesity.* Front. Endocrinol. (Lausanne), 2017. 8: p. 54.

125.	Lee, W., *The CEACAM1 expression is decreased in the liver of severely obese patients with or without diabetes.* Diagn. Pathol., 2011. 6: p. 40.

126.	Xu, E., et al., *Targeted disruption of carcinoembryonic antigen-related cell adhesion molecule 1 promotes diet-induced hepatic steatosis and insulin resistance.* Endocrinology, 2009. 150: p. 3503-3512.

127.	DeAngelis, A.M., et al., *Carcinoembryonic antigen-related cell adhesion molecule 1: a link between insulin and lipid metabolism.* Diabetes, 2008. 57(9): p. 2296-303.

128.	Poy, M.N., et al., *CEACAM1 regulates insulin clearance in liver.* Nat. Genet., 2002. 30(3): p. 270-6.

129.    Najjar, S.M., et al., *Insulin acutely decreases hepatic fatty acid synthase activity.* Cell Metab., 2005. 2(1): p. 43-53.

130.    Najjar, S.M. and L. Russo, *CEACAM1 loss links inflammation to insulin resistance in obesity and non-alcoholic steatohepatitis (NASH).* Semin. Immunopathol., 2014. 36(1): p. 55-71.

131.    Najjar, S.M., et al., *Ceacam1 deletion causes vascular alterations in large vessels.* Am. J. Physiol. Endocrinol. Metab., 2013. 305(4): p. E519-29.

132.    Ghosh, S., et al., *Mice with null mutation of Ceacam I develop nonalcoholic steatohepatitis.* Hepat. Med: Res. Evidence, 2010. 2010(2): p. 69-78.

133.    Ghadieh, H.E., et al., *Loss of Hepatic Carcinoembryonic Antigen-Related Cell Adhesion Molecule 1 Links Nonalcoholic Steatohepatitis to Atherosclerosis.* Hepatol. Commun., 2020. 4(11): p. 1591-1609.

134.    Horst, A.K., et al., *CEACAM1 in Liver Injury, Metabolic and Immune Regulation.* Int. J. Mol. Sci., 2018. 19(10).

135.    Al-Share, Q.Y., et al., *Forced Hepatic Overexpression of CEACAM1 Curtails Diet-Induced Insulin Resistance.* Diabetes, 2015. 64(8): p. 2780-90.

136.    Tacke, F. and H.W. Zimmermann, *Macrophage heterogeneity in liver injury and fibrosis.* J. Hepatol., 2014. 60(5): p. 1090-6.

137.    Adelaja, A. and A. Hoffmann, *Signaling Crosstalk Mechanisms That May Fine-Tune Pathogen-Responsive NFkappaB.* Front. Immunol., 2019. 10: p. 433.

138.    Suryavanshi, S.V. and Y.A. Kulkarni, *NF-kappabeta: A Potential Target in the Management of Vascular Complications of Diabetes.* Front. Pharmacol., 2017. 8: p. 798.

139.    Gregor, M.F. and G.S. Hotamisligil, *Inflammatory mechanisms in obesity.* Ann Rev Immunol, 2011. 29: p. 415-45.

140.    Abdel-Razzak, Z., et al., *Determination of interleukin-4-responsive region in the human cytochrome P450 2E1 gene promoter.* Biochem, Pharmacol,, 2004. 68(7): p. 1371-81.

141.    Mari, M., et al., *Mitochondrial free cholesterol loading sensitizes to TNF- and Fas-mediated steatohepatitis.* Cell Metab, 2006. 4: p. 185-198.

142.    Cai, D., et al., *Local and systemic insulin resistance resulting from hepatic activation of IKK-beta and NF-kappaB.* Nat. Med., 2005. 11(2): p. 183-90.

143.    Manicassamy, S., et al., *Protein kinase C-theta-mediated signals enhance CD4+ T cell survival by up-regulating Bcl-xL.* J Immunol, 2006. 176: p. 6709-6716.

144.    Nagarajan, R.P., et al., *Repression of transforming-growth-factor-beta-mediated transcription by nuclear factor kappaB.* Biochem. J., 2000. 348 Pt 3: p. 591-6.

145.    Russo, L., et al., *Liver-specific rescuing of CEACAM1 reverses endothelial and cardiovascular abnormalities in male mice with null deletion of Ceacam1 gene.* Mol. Metab., 2018. 9: p. 98-113.

146.    Mahmoud, A.M., et al., *Hyperinsulinemia augments endothelin-1 protein expression and impairs vasodilation of human skeletal muscle arterioles.* Physiol. Rep., 2016. 4(16).

147. van Uden, P., N.S. Kenneth, and S. Rocha, *Regulation of hypoxia-inducible factor-1alpha by NF-kappaB.* Biochem. J., 2008. 412(3): p. 477-84.

148. Au, P.Y., et al., *The oncogene PDGF-B provides a key switch from cell death to survival induced by TNF.* Oncogene, 2005. 24(19): p. 3196-205.

149. Wan, J., et al., *LC3-associated phagocytosis in myeloid cells, a fireman that restrains inflammation and liver fibrosis, via immunoreceptor inhibitory signaling.* Autophagy, 2020. 16(8): p. 1526-1528.

150. Musso, G., R. Gambino, and M. Cassader, *Cholesterol metabolism and the pathogenesis of non-alcoholic steatohepatitis.* Prog. Lipid Res., 2013. 52(1): p. 175-91.

151. Carter-Kent, C., N.N. Zein, and A.E. Feldstein, *Cytokines in the pathogenesis of fatty liver and disease progression to steatohepatitis: implications for treatment.* Am J Gastroenterol, 2008. 103: p. 1036-1042.

152. Friedman, S.L., *Mechanisms of hepatic fibrogenesis.* Gastroenterology, 2008. 134(6): p. 1655-69.

153. Yokota, T., et al., *Role of protein kinase C on the expression of platelet-derived growth factor and endothelin-1 in the retina of diabetic rats and cultured retinal capillary pericytes.* Diabetes, 2003. 52(3): p. 838-45.

154. Nakamura, K., et al., *Hepatic CEACAM1 expression indicates donor liver quality and prevents early transplantation injury.* J. Clin. Invest., 2020. 130(5): p. 2689-2704.

155. Musso, G., et al., *Pioglitazone for advanced fibrosis in nonalcoholic steatohepatitis: New evidence, new challenges.* Hepatology, 2017. 65(3): p. 1058-1061.

156. Ghadieh, H.E., et al., *Exenatide induces carcinoembryonic antigen-related cell adhesion molecule 1 expression to prevent hepatic steatosis.* Hepatol. Commun., 2018. 2(1): p. 35-47.

157. Hess, P.L., et al., *The Metabolic Syndrome and Risk of Sudden Cardiac Death: The Atherosclerosis Risk in Communities Study.* J Am Heart Assoc, 2017. 6(8).

158. Wang, T., et al., *NASH in Nondiabetic Endocrine Disorders.* Metab Syndr Relat Disord, 2018. 16(7): p. 315-320.

159. Ong, J.P. and Z.M. Younossi, *Epidemiology and natural history of NAFLD and NASH.* Clin Liver Dis, 2007. 11(1): p. 1-16, vii.

160. Weber, C. and H. Noels, *Atherosclerosis: current pathogenesis and therapeutic options.* Nat Med, 2011. 17(11): p. 1410-22.

161. Russo, L., et al., *Liver-specific rescuing of CEACAM1 reverses endothelial and cardiovascular abnormalities in male mice with null deletion of Ceacam1 gene.* Mol Metab, 2018. 9: p. 98-113.